HARD-EARNED LIVES

HARD-EARNED LIVES
*Accounts of Health and Illness
from East London*

Jocelyn Cornwell

Tavistock Publications
London and New York

First published in 1984 by
Tavistock Publications Ltd.
11 New Fetter Lane, London EC4P 4EE
Published in the USA by
Tavistock Publications
in association with Methuen Inc.
733 Third Avenue, New York, NY 10017

Typeset by Graphicraft Typesetters Ltd., Hong Kong
Printed in Great Britain by
J.W. Arrowsmith Ltd, Bristol

British Library Cataloguing in Publication Data

Cornwell, Jocelyn
  Hard-earned lives.
  1. Medical care—Great Britain—Public
  opinion—Case studies   2. Public opinion
  —England—London—Case studies
  I. Title
  362.1′0722   RA395.G6

  ISBN 0-422-78580-6

Library of Congress Cataloging in Publication Data

Cornwell, Jocelyn.
  Hard-earned lives.

  Based on the author's thesis (Ph. D.—London University)
  Bibliography: p.
  Includes indexes.
  1. Health attitudes—England—London–Case studies.
2. Labor and laboring classes—Health and hygiene—
England—London—Case studies.   I. Title.
RA488.L8C67 1984   362.1′042   84-8808
ISBN 0-422-78580-6

Contents

Acknowledgements

This book is based on the work for a Phd. thesis in the Department of Geography and Earth Science at Queen Mary College, London University. I should like to thank all the members of the Health Research Group in the Geography Department for their interest in the project, and especially Professor David Smith, Dr John Eyles, and Dr Kevin Woods for reading it in draft form. David Smith supervised the work and I feel very grateful to him, not only for giving comments and criticisms which have always been helpful, but also for the encouragement and practical help he has provided at times when it was very sorely needed.

Dr Vieda Skultans of the Department of Mental Health at Bristol University acted as external supervisor to the thesis, and I should like to thank her for taking on that role. The fact that she was there to be consulted and was reading the various drafts of the work gave me confidence about the direction of the project which I would otherwise have lacked. I should also like to thank Professor Margaret Stacey for her helpful comments.

There is a very large number of people who, in one way or another, have helped me complete the work for this book, all of whom I should like to thank, especially: Rel Constantine, Brian and Marianne Cornwell, Georgie and Sam Fogg, Dave Leon, Colin MacCabe, Martha McIntyre, Linda Marks, Patrick O'Neill, Rosie Parker, Ruthie Petrie, Sara Rance, Alastair Reid, Holly Sutherland, and Sophie Watson.

I am very grateful to Audrey Kinsella for typing the manuscript and for giving it so much of her time and attention. The interest which she and Pat O'Neill showed in the work in its final stages has been tremendously supportive.

Barbora Hájková designed the family trees and Lynne Fraser and Richard West in the Cartographic Unit at Queen Mary College laid them out; my thanks to them all for their technical assistance.

Finally, and most important of all, I am grateful to everyone who took part in the interviews, and especially to Kathleen Read, Alice Moss, and her friend A. E. In order to disguise people's identities I have given them all different names and made slight alterations to the details of their personal lives and histories which are of little or no consequence for the substance of the text. I am indebted to everyone who was interviewed, not only for co-operating in the research but for making that part of it so enjoyable.

Jocelyn Cornwell
April 1984.

1 *The Study: Research Methods and Theoretical Considerations*

Introduction

This book is an enquiry into the lives of twenty-four people – fifteen women and nine men – who live in East London. Its chief concern is with their commonsense ideas and theories about health, illness, and health services, but it is based on the assumption that if we are to understand the significance they attach to this, as to any area of their lives, then we have to consider its place in the context of their lives as a whole.

The book has more in common with social anthropology than with other disciplines in the social sciences, in so far as the emphasis in social anthropology is all the time on the whole and on the links between apparently discrete areas of social life. In social anthropology the object of study is social processes and there is an attempt to grasp how the different elements in the life of a people, whether it is a tribe, a village, or a residential neighbourhood, are integrated together. In contrast, in the other disciplines in the social sciences, i.e., in medical sociology, social psychology, and medical geography, there is a tendency for matters relating to health to be separated out as subjects that can be investigated in isolation from other aspects of social life.

Perhaps the most useful way to describe the research method adopted in the study is to call it a case study which attempts to give a theoretical as well as a descriptive account of its case material (Mitchell 1983:195). The twenty four cases (individuals) on which the study is based were not randomly selected and cannot therefore be regarded as 'typical' or 'representative' in the statistical sense. They are however 'typical' in the colloquial meaning of the word: their lives faithfully reflect the history of social and economic life in East London over the past eighty or more years. The families of the people involved in the study have formed and reformed in the appalling housing conditions in East

London before the war and under the impact of the Blitz and the slum clearance and reconstruction which followed after it; the men and women in these families do the jobs that the local labour market makes available to them as the men and women in previous generations in their families did before them; whether or not they receive help when they are ill, as well as what kind of help they receive, is bound up with the particular pattern of provision of health services in this part of London.

The case study approach is particularly suited to the purpose of the enquiry because it permits a level of detail and thoroughness in the observation of cases which is unique. The researcher is able to get to know the people in the study individually and to know the quality of their relationships with other people and can see how, even within the same family, there are differences between individuals which occur because of the choices each of them makes for themselves. This is not meant to imply that people have a great deal of choice about the conditions in which they lead their lives – it is quite clear in the discussions to follow that the people involved in this study have had very few choices – but that as a method of research the case study is unlikely to reduce its subjects to ciphers, figures so socially determined that they lack the ability to take an active part in the process of their own lives.

It is also useful to draw attention to the similarities between this enquiry and some studies of 'community'. The people involved in the study all live in one area and most of them know one another, either because they are related or because they are friends or neighbours. The study has the difficulty, common in community studies generally, of knowing where the line should be drawn between what is particular to the community and what is part of belonging to the wider society (see Dennis, Henriques and Slaughter 1969: 7). Like most community studies it does not attempt to solve the problem directly. It makes the basic assumption that the 'external factors' are there and are integral to everything which takes place in the community but, rather than attempting to make the connections between the two explicit, it focusses on what is unique about East London in terms of its housing, the local labour market, the shifts in populations and so on.

In the early stages of planning the research the concept of the 'informal social network' figured largely. Since the aim of the study was to understand the lives of its subjects as fully as possible, it was obviously important to establish who they saw regularly and what kind of relationships they had with other people. There is a vast literature on informal social networks in social anthopology (see Barnes 1969a; 1969b; Mitchell 1969), in the sociology of the family (see Bott 1957; Harris 1969) and in the sociology of medicine (see Freidson 1961; 1970; Kadushin 1966; Horwitz 1977; Finlayson and McEwen 1977; Pilisuk and Froland 1978; Price 1981) in which it is frequently, and regretfully noted that, for practical reasons, most studies of informal social networks have relied on only one source for their information about a whole network of social relationships. There is a plethora of 'ego-centred' network studies (Horwitz 1977) which use one person or – in Bott's case – one couple as the source for information about relationships in the network as a whole, but very few studies which make use of a number of accounts from different sources in the same network. In view of this it seemed desirable to break with tradition and, acknowledging the practical limitations, to make a study of one or possibly two social networks using information from more than one source.

The research for the book took place in three stages, referred to as the pilot and the first and second stages of interviewing. In the pilot and the first stage of interviewing, people were recruited to the study through their informal social networks. The pilot study involved six people (see *Figure 1.2*) – four women and two men – in three separate households, all of whom knew one another and were connected through a network of friendships and neighbourliness. The first set of interviews involved seven people (see *Figure 1.2*) – six women and one man – in six separate households all of whom belonged to the same extended family: the Davies's. In the second and final set of interviews, it was decided to abandon *the principle* of recruiting people in the same social networks because, on balance, it seemed that *as a principle* it was no longer of practical benefit to the research.

The chief advantage of this method of recruitment had turned out to be the personal introductions that people in a network of relationships could provide to other people in their network. Having personal introductions made the initial contact with people much easier and helped to make the atmosphere surrounding the interviews much less formal than it might otherwise have been, and this, in turn, made it possible to obtain 'private' as well as 'public' accounts of the subjects which were broached. (For a discussion of public vs. private accounts and the difference between them see below pp. 11–17.) However, for the specific purposes of this research, the term 'social network' had proved something of a misnomer. The importance of 'the network' as a medium for the exchange of ideas, advice, and information about health and health services seemed to have been greatly exaggerated. There were exchanges of this kind, but they rarely involved more than two or three people, and never the entire network.

More important was the fact that from the data which had been gathered from the pilot and first stage of interviews, it was clear that it was women much more than men who were actively involved in the relationships that held the network together. The 'network' was much less a network than it was a series of relationships between women. By the end of the first stage it was apparent from the interviews which had been completed that employment outside the home and the sexual division of labour inside the home were subjects that needed to be further researched and, in order to do this, I needed to interview more men. Being female myself, and given what has already been said about the active relationships in the network involving women, it was relatively easy for me to be taken up by the women and to be passed from one to the next. However, once I was involved in this way with the women I found it very difficult to make contact with men. In the Davies family the women I interviewed were not at all enthusiastic about asking their husbands to take part in the study and I was reluctant to risk jeopardizing the relationships I had established with them by becoming insistent.

In the second and final stage of the research I decided not to recruit people in the same social network but to concentrate instead on finding men who would agree to be interviewed. The way I achieved this was by going to a meeting of the local Resident's Association on the estate where I had already interviewed some people and asking for volunteers. No volunteers came forward and I then approached individual men on its Committee (which had endorsed my request for volunteers) and asked them if they would agree to be interviewed.

Figures 1.1–4 provide a very brief guide to the people who took part in the study and their relationships to each other:

The pilot study (Figure 1.1)

Six people were involved in the pilot study:

Jeannie Moss and her daughter, Alice Moss

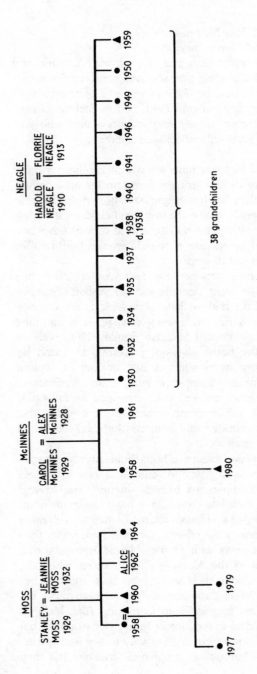

MOSS

STANLEY = JEANNIE
MOSS   MOSS
1929   1932

● = ▲   ▲   ALICE   ●
1958   1960   1962   1964

▲   ●
1977   1979

McINNES

CAROL = ALEX
McINNES   McINNES
1929   1928

▲   ●
1958   1961

▲
1980

NEAGLE

HAROLD = FLORRIE
NEAGLE   NEAGLE
1910   1913

●   ●   ●   ▲   ▲   ▲   ●   ●   ▲   ●   ▲
1930 1932 1934 1935 1937 1938 1940 1941 1946 1949 1950 1959
                         d.1938

38 grandchildren

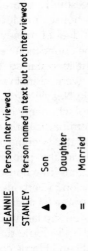

JEANNIE   Person interviewed
STANLEY   Person named in text but not interviewed

▲   Son
●   Daughter
=   Married

Figure 1.1   The Pilot Study

5

Carol and Alex McInnes
Harold and Florrie Neagle

A local insurance agent gave me Jeannie Moss's name and address on the understanding that she was someone he found friendly and thought would be likely to agree to be interviewed. Jeannie was the very first person I contacted in Bethnal Green, and it is no exaggeration to say that everyone else who was interviewed became involved – directly or indirectly – because of her.

Jeannie and Carol McInnes have known each other for thirty years and have more or less brought their families up together. Both women are in their late forties and have grown-up children; both are grandmothers as well as having adult children still living at home. They have always been close and at various times one or other of them has taken care of the children in both families whilst the other went out to work.

Despite the closeness between the two women, their two households are very different. Jeannie and her husband Stan live under the same roof but have as little as possible to do with one another. The house is run on Jeannie's wage as a part-time receptionist in a local hospital because Stanley Moss will not contribute towards the house-keeping, preferring to spend his earnings on expensive items such as his car and the colour television which dominates their small living room. In contrast, Carol and Alex McInnes present their marriage as extremely successful. Both are in full time employment and it is evident that their house, newly decorated and very comfortable, has had a great deal of money spent on it.

The connection between these two households and the Neagles originally occurred because Alex McInnes and Harold Neagle who were drinking companions became friends. Harold and Florrie Neagle are in their late sixties; they have twelve children, nine of whom are married and have children of their own. Neither of them particularly enjoys the other's company and, rather than spend the evening indoors with Florrie, Harold is usually out, either in the pub or in the McInnes's living room where he entertains the household with stories of his past and watches television. Everyone in all three families knows each other but only some of them are friends. Both Carol and Alex McInnes attended the last wedding in the Neagle family, for example, but Carol and Florrie do not go out of their way to see each other. Harold and Florrie call themselves 'rough nuts', meaning that they are not afraid of physical violence or of the police; Alice Moss described the Neagles as 'one of the local mafias'.

The first set of interviews: the Davies family (Figure 1.2)

My first contact with the Davies family was through Kathleen Read, who lives in the same street as the Mosses and the McInneses and whom Alice Moss suggested I contact. Kathleen is fifty and has been married and widowed twice. She has four children – a son and two daughters by her first marriage, all of whom are now grown-up, and a much younger daughter by her second marriage. Stan Flowers, Kathleen's second husband was interviewed once for the study; he was a very quiet and shy man and found being interviewed a torture. A year after the interview, during a brief illness which initially appeared to be 'flu, Stan was diagnosed as having cancer and nine months later he died. Kathleen now lives on her own with her daughter, who is seven.

Kathleen's two elder daughters, Sharon and Joanne, both of whom I interviewed, live within walking distance of their mother and rely on her for help with their own children. This is particularly true of Joanne who is a single mother and lives on her own with her three young children.

Kathleen herself originally came from a family of eleven children, four boys and seven girls. One of her brothers died in infancy and another died more recently, in 1976, of cancer. Four of her sisters have moved away from the East End and all that is left of the family locally are her two sisters, Joan and Mary (interviewed twice and three times respectively), her parents, Nellie (interviewed once) and Arthur Davies, and the two remaining brothers.

The second set of interviews (Figures 1.3 and 1.4)

The people who took part in the second and final stage of the research can be usefully divided into those who are part of the Scott family (*Figure 1.3*) and the rest, who are neighbours on the estate where the Moss and McInnes households and Kathleen Read all live (*Figure 1.4*). I initially met William Cox who was representing his street at the Residents' Association meeting. William agreed to be interviewed and to introduce me to his wife,

7

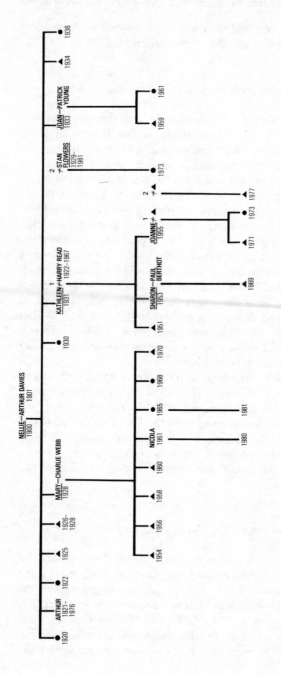

MARY   Person interviewed

CHARLIE Person named in text but not interviewed

▲ Son

● Daughter

— Married

† Marriage over

1 First marriage

2 Second marriage

Figure 1.2 The Davies Family Tree

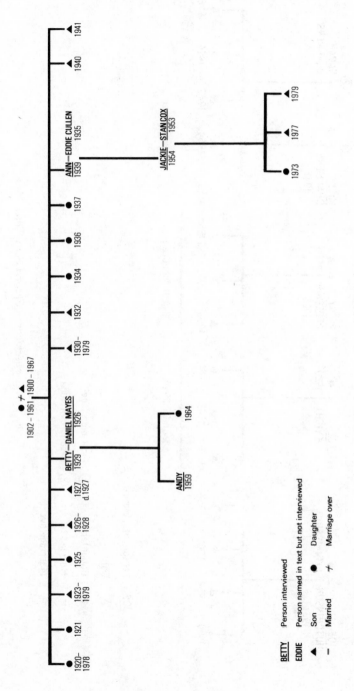

Figure 1.3 The Scott Family Tree

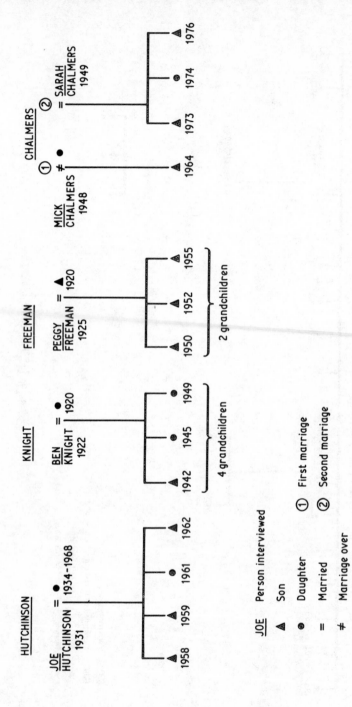

Figure 1.4 Households in Second Set of Interviews

HUTCHINSON

JOE HUTCHINSON 1931 = ● 1934–1968

△ 1958 △ 1959 ● 1961 △ 1962

KNIGHT

BEN KNIGHT 1922 = ● 1920

△ 1942 ● 1945 ● 1949

4 grandchildren

FREEMAN

PEGGY FREEMAN 1925 = △ 1920

△ 1950 △ 1952 △ 1955

2 grandchildren

CHALMERS

MICK CHALMERS 1948

① # ●

△ 1964

② = SARAH CHALMERS 1949

△ 1973 ● 1974 △ 1976

JOE   Person interviewed

△   Son

●   Daughter

=   Married

Marriage over

①   First marriage

②   Second marriage

Jackie, who also agreed. Through Jackie I was able to arrange interviews with her mother Ann Cullen, who visits her every day and whom I met in her house, and with her aunt, uncle, and cousin who live close-by. Joe Hutchinson, Ben Knight, Peggy Freeman, and Mick Chalmers were all at the Residents' Association meeting, and all of them agreed to be interviewed as did Sarah Chalmers, Mick's wife, whom I met later. Ben Knight and Peggy Freeman were unable to get their partners to agree to take part in the research, and Joe Hutchinson is a widower and lives alone with his four teen-age children.

All the interviews for the study were recorded on tape and took place in people's homes: in all, a total of seventy hours interviewing was recorded and notes of a further sixty hours spent in people's homes are also available. The majority of the interviews were conducted in private, away from the rest of the household, but there were odd occasions in the interviews with both Sarah and Mick Chalmers and with Daniel Mayes, when someone else was in the room for at least part of an interview. Everyone in the study knew I was a student and gave 'being of help' to me in my studies as their reason for agreeing to the interviews. Later, when I apologised for taking up their time their reaction was usually 'it's got to be done', as if the research was now a fact of *their* lives as well as mine. The explanation I gave for what I was doing was that I wanted to study local people's experience of health and illness and health services and that in order to do that properly, I wanted to enquire into other areas of their lives which were not directly connected with their health, specifying family history, education, employment, and housing.

The interviews were constructed around a schedule of topics. They included some standard questions which were put to everyone and also questions developed specifically for each individual each time he or she was interviewed, which made use of information from earlier interviews with them and with other people.

Interpreting the findings

One of the themes that the book uses the interview material to explore concerns the different types of account people give of health matters in particular, but also of themselves and their experience more generally. It argues that what people say, and how they say it, varies according to who they are talking to and the circumstances in which they find themselves. In the course of the research, the same people gave accounts of events in their own pasts which were substantially different from the accounts they had given of the same events on previous occasions. It seemed to me that these variations were not tricks of memory, they occurred because of changes in the relationship they had with me, the interviewer, and were also related to different techniques of interviewing. In the chapters to follow, the terms 'public' and 'private accounts' are used to distinguish differences in the way people talked in the interviews, and the origins and meanings of these terms will briefly be explained.

My experience of doing the interviews and establishing relationships with the various people taking part in the study was comparable to the account Oakley has given of her experience interviewing women for her study of childbirth and the transition to motherhood (Oakley 1981). Like her, and unlike the one-off interviews which are the norm in standard surveys, I interviewed the same people repeatedly; furthermore, I interviewed different people in the same household repeatedly. I shared Oakley's view of the techniques and methods of conducting interviews recommended in some textbooks (see Selltiz *et al.* 1965; Sjoberg and Nett 1968; Richardson 1965; Galtung 1969) as basically techniques and methods of manipulating people and calculatedly treating them as objects in order to get what one wants out of them (Oakley 1981: 33). Apart from considering, as she does, that it is unethical to treat people like this, I felt it would be an unproductive path to follow. In asking people to take part in the study I was asking them to give me hours of their time, spread over weeks and even months, and in most cases I was also asking them to furnish me with introductions to their relatives and friends. It seemed highly implausible that they would agree to any of this if they sensed they were being used, so my priority in composing the schedules for the interviews and interviewing people was, as much as possible, to take my cue from them, to let them direct the course of the interview and to follow their interest in the topics I proposed to them.

Oakley's solution to the ethical difficulties involved in using human subjects for research purposes is to rely on the concept of 'sisterhood'. She maintains that 'sisterhood' can provide a vehicle for overcoming inequalities between the interviewer and the interviewee (provided of course that both are women), and says she appealed to what is common to women and to their life experience in building relationships with the women she interviewed. To some extent this applies to the relationships I developed with the women in the study. It was noticeable that the atmosphere in the interviews with all the women was easier and the interviews were accomplished with less difficulty than the interviews with the men: there was a familiarity between myself and the women, and an understanding of how to approach each other which did not occur with the men. The men – quite literally – did not know how to talk to me: they did not know whether or not to swear or tell jokes and also had very little idea what to say about personal matters.

However, in her discussion of 'sisterhood', Oakley skates over one very important aspect of the research process, which is the significance of the differences in social class and educational background which are so common in relationships between academic researchers and their research subjects. In this enquiry, the men's awkwardness about swearing was only one of a number of indicators of the effects these differences had on the interviews with both sexes. To give an example: in the first interview with Jeannie Moss I asked her how she got on with her neighbours, and she replied that they were all very friendly and there was no-one in the street who would not lend a helping hand if it was needed. Weeks later, and on the occasion of my sixth visit to the house to interview Jeannie's daughter Alice, Alice and Jeannie together described with immense pleasure and humour the verbal and physical fights that take place in their street, with neighbours striking one another and calling the police to each other's doors, and families in the street who have been feuding for years.

It is arguable that the polite responses people give to questions asked by someone whom they hardly know are an indication of the good manners that conventionally mark social distance. Thus, at the first meeting, Jeannie Moss – wanting to be polite and to give a good impression – avoided mentioning aspects of community life that might have seemed rude or undesirable. In any new social situation where people are unsure of their ground, they become acutely concerned with making sure they know what is going on and with managing their own part in it correctly (Goffman 1959: 241). The activities of 'managing appearances' and 'controlling information', according to Goffman, are continuous elements of all social interaction. But in novel situations and *especially* in situations which are unfamiliar *and* unequal, they are at the forefront of awareness.

The research interview is invariably a situation that is new and unfamiliar for research subjects and, classically, a situation in which they feel and are made to feel unequal. For Sennett (1980), the 'expert' is the modern face of authority and 'experts' are people in autonomous occupations, occupations that require them to be trained and to train themselves. The quintessential autonomous expert is the doctor, but academics also fit the description perfectly. In this study, the fact that I am middle class, have had further education, and am female, in a part of London where it is unusual for people to have been educated beyond secondary level and to have professional occupations, and especially unusual for a woman, made me into a kind of expert for the people I was interviewing. In East London, most middle class people are, after all, experts of one kind or another.

In an interview, which involves nothing but talking, language and the content of what is said, become all-important. The following extract from one of the later interviews with Kathleen Read illustrates how much using the 'right' words and saying the 'right' things matters in this kind of circumstance. Kathleen had been talking about her feeling of being 'tongue-tied' in front of doctors and was explaining why it was that she had a similar feeling with her daughter's probation officer:

KR: 'Someone that I find I think it's something of importance, probably it's because, in me mind's eye, I'm not educated all that well and I'm frightened and I am going to say the wrong words, probably. I don't know, but I did, I used to get that sort of feeling when I went to see her.'

JC: 'Do you think that's something they bring to it, or is it something you create?'

KR: 'No, I should imagine it's meself, really. Probably getting meself worked up for no reason at all really. Wondering if I'm going to say the right thing or put me foot wrong. Or, or even if, like the other night we had a woman come round about the houses, I'm pretty sure I was saying everything back to front. Now I knew the woman was coming from the GLC, but she was sort of pumping the questions at me, and I thought, well, how do you answer them, you know? And I mean, I was telling her about me roof and I don't think she wrote that down and things like that. I was trying to sort of . . . I was getting meself into such a state, I don't think she got half the things down that poor woman wanted anyway. And yet I knew she was coming. Probably it's being strangers . . . I don't know.'

JC: 'Is it that what you're talking about is important to you? Or is it because they're important people?'

KR: 'As far as I'm concerned it's supposed to be an important issue, really. Isn't it? Seeing as it's to do with your house, if you think it's in good condition, poor. I couldn't even tell the woman if I thought this house was a fair conditioned house, a poor conditioned house, or a reasonable. I turned round and said, "Well, I don't know".'

JC: 'That's what she asked you?'

KR: 'Yes. She said, "What condition would you say your house was in?". Well, to me, it's like a shambles really, for what wants doing to it, but when you think round, there's other houses in a worse state than what yours is, and there's some that's better. So I said, "Just put down fair", but no doubt if they checked over it they would have turned round and said to them it's a poor house really. I can't think for meself at times, when people put different questions to me.'

Another way to describe the phenomenon of managing one's appearance, is to say that people cope with situations which are entirely new to them and where they are uncertain of their own position in relation to others by putting on their 'best face' (Laslett and Rapoport 1975). This does not necessarily mean that they are 'dissimulating or attempting to mislead the interviewer', but what they are doing is reproducing the 'culturally normative pattern' (Laslett and Rapoport 1975: 973), or – as it is termed here – sticking to the relative security offered by 'public accounts'.

Public accounts are sets of meanings in common social currency that reproduce and legitimate the assumptions people take for granted about the nature of social reality. There is a public account of most subjects which occur with any regularity in everyday conversations, the point being that in sticking to the public account of whatever it is they are discussing – whether it is work, or money, husbands, mothers, children, or the local doctor – the person doing the talking can be sure that whatever they say will be acceptable to other people. Public accounts, in Douglas's words, conform to 'least common denominator morality' (Douglas 1971: 242).

The opposite of the public account is the 'private account' which expresses what Douglas describes as the way in which a person 'would respond if thinking only what he and the people he knows directly would think and do' (Douglas 1971: 242). Private accounts spring directly from personal experience and from the thoughts and feelings accompanying it.

In the interviews, the differences between the two types of account were usually apparent. Most of the first interviews with each person were mainly taken up with public accounts, and it was usually only in later interviews and often when a subject had already been broached once, that people gave private accounts. It was noticeable too that the accounts people gave varied according to whether they had been asked a direct question – when they responded with public accounts – or invited to tell a story – in which case they might give private accounts. I would argue that the explanation for this variation is that a subtle shift of power takes place in the relationship between the interviewer and the interviewee according to whether the interviewer is asking questions or encouraging the other person to tell stories. In the first instance the relationship between the two is controlled by the interviewer; in the second it is more controlled by the story-teller. In the course of a single interview, the person being asked questions and answering them seemed reminded of the unnaturalness of what they were doing, talking about themselves to a stranger who was making a study of them. But when they were telling stories, their attention was focussed on the story and the events it contained rather than the audience, and they shifted into a different and less self-conscious way of talking about the thoughts and feelings associated with their experience.

It seems likely that differences of class and education will always be associated in some degree with the 'best face' phenomenon (Laslett and Rapoport 1975: 970) and therefore with the production of public accounts. In standard surveys variations of the kind that have been outlined are treated as a 'problem of bias', and interviewers are trained in techniques designed to 'overcome' them. Here however, this is accepted as a part of the social reality which is being investigated and as a valuable source of data concerning the way people in the study conduct themselves with strangers and in cross-class relationships. This data is of course particularly pertinent to the discussion of their relationships with doctors and other health workers which follows (see Chapter 7).

To return very briefly to Oakley: she maintains that the ethical position for the interviewer/researcher to adopt in relation to the subjects of her research is that she should see herself as a 'data recording instrument for those whose lives are being researched', rather than a 'data collecting instrument for other researchers' (Oakley 1981: 49). She does not mention the 'best face' phenomenon, nor does she comment on the distinction between public and private accounts, perhaps because there were not these kind of variations in the interviews she did with women. Is it perhaps that there are no public accounts of uniquely female experiences? This seems unlikely. The women in this study had public as well as private accounts of childbirth and the care of young children, the two areas of Oakley's concern.

The interviewer cannot simply be a 'recording instrument' because who she is, what she is like, and the relationship she has with the interviewee affects the content of the interviews. This observation is fundamental to the interpretation of all the material from the interviews in this study. The interviews contain public as well as private accounts of everything, of work, husbands, mothers, children, housing, doctors, illness, and so on. The significance of the difference between the two is one of the major themes explored in the book, and is also integral to the other major theme which concerns the part medicine plays in relation to the whole area of health and illness. For, unlike most of the topics mentioned above, i.e. work, husbands, mothers, etc., our culture assumes that health is a subject for experts, something only doctors really know about, and this has a profound effect on the relationship 'ordinary people', people who are not medically qualified, have with it. The effect on the interviews was that in their public accounts of health-related matters, people made sure that what they said was not only non-controversial, and thus likely to be acceptable, but that it conformed with their notion of the 'medical point of view'.

This brings us directly to the second of the two major themes in the book, which is that of the relationship between medicine and the medical profession on the one hand, and society – 'ordinary people' – on the other. Exactly what kind of role medicine plays in society is a question that has preoccupied medical sociologists ever since Parsons originally chose medicine to illustrate the part played by 'institutions of social control' in maintaining the social order (Parsons 1951). Each school of social thought has its own interpretation of that role and it is not possible to do justice to the very extensive literature on this subject in this brief discussion.

17

However, although the interpretations of the way in which medicine functions as an institution of social control differ, Parsons's original contention that medicine *is* an institution of social control has remained central to the sociological account of medicine's role in society and to the way in which sociologists have interpreted the relationship between the medical profession and the 'ordinary people' who are its patients.

In this study, the concept of medicalization is put forward as an alternative to the definition of medicine as an institution of social control, the latter being considered unsatisfactory for a number of reasons. First, there are no empirical grounds for characterizing medicine simply as 'an institution' (Freidson 1970; Strong 1979a). Medicine is a hierarchy of different specialist groups with conflicting interests, and the medical profession is divided along lines of sex, age, and race, as well as between doctors with different styles of medical practice and medical beliefs.

Second, all the major schools of sociological thought represented in medical sociology focus on the *ideological* sway medicine has over everything associated with health and illness, to the exclusion of all other considerations. In doing so, they offer accounts of medicine's social role that are 'idealist', i.e., they over-estimate the ideological importance of medical practice and under-estimate its actual achievements. These analyses ignore the practical benefits which, in very many instances, medicine offers patients and are therefore unable to explain why patients should actively seek out medical treatment.

The third point concerns the view of the patient that is associated with the definition of medicine as an institution of social control. Each school of thought in medical sociology has its own analysis of the patient: the structural-functionalist view is not that of the radical theorist, which is different again from the view of the interpretive sociologist. The classic structural-functionalist position (Parsons 1951) defines medicine as a science and contrasts it with lay theorizing which is unscientific. Science is associated with rationality, objectivity, and everything modern; non-science (superstition) with irrationality, subjectivity, and tradition. Medicine is used as a yardstick against which lay concepts of health and illness are measured, with the result that patients' reactions to illness are characterized as (over-) emotional, subjective, irrational, and ignorant (Parsons 1951: 441–43; Freidson 1970: 288–300).

The premise from which radical, or conflict, theorists work is that the interests of doctors and patients are antagonistic and that it is the task of the critic or the sociologist to ally him or herself with patients. (The reference is to 'critics or sociologists' because the radicals include Illich (1976) who is probably best regarded as a 'theoretician of industrialism' (Navarro 1977: 106), as well as writers who identify themselves more with Marxism or with feminism (see Navarro 1977; Ehrenreich and Ehrenreich 1978; Waitzkin 1979; Ehrenreich and English 1973; Barrett and Roberts 1978) than with sociology.) However, the radical analysis of medicine as an ideologically oppressive institution leads to an analysis of patients which is curiously paradoxical. Radical theorists want to be 'on the side of the patient' but they regard patients' statements about their own health and needs for health care (especially if they want more medical intervention and treatment) as ideologically suspect, and patients themselves as the victims of 'false consciousness'.

In theory, structural functionalism and radical theory are profoundly different: in practice they amount to an analysis which invalidates 'ordinary people's' view of health, illness, and health services and which, incidentally, has at least until recently discouraged medical sociologists from taking patients' views seriously.

There is a third school of interpretive medical sociologists whose approach is more conducive to the study of patients' points of view than either of the two approaches which have been outlined, but there are severe practical difficulties in moving it for the purposes of empirical research. The interpretive paradigm rejects epistemological hierarchies – i.e. Parsons's science/non-science distinction – (see Dingwall 1976; Voysey 1975; Sudnow 1967) and manages to acknowledge the existence of medical power without turning patients into passive, acquiescent, or dependent victims. Patients, all social actors, are seen as people who actively and creatively produce and reproduce the meanings that sustain their social world in every moment of their interactions with other people. The approach leads more readily to serious treatment of lay concepts of health and illness, but the range of empirical work it has actually generated has been limited to studies of disability and handicap (Davis 1960; 1963; Voysey 1975) and patients in medical settings (Sudnow 1967; Glaser and Strauss 1965; Davis and Horobin 1977; Cowie 1976). This limitation has partly occurred because of the methodological difficulties involved in extending the approach to non-medical settings.

The basic methodology of the interpretive sociologies is personal observation, with varying degrees of participation on the part of the researcher. It is a great deal easier to be an observer in an institutional setting such as a hospital ward or an out-patient clinic, than in a private setting such as someone's home, or a pub or a family gathering. The researcher interested in producing an interpretive account of lay concepts of health and illness would have to be able to observe all the places, public as well as private, in which people talk about their health (Voysey 1975: 74). Not only would it be difficult to accomplish this in private settings without altering the subjects' behaviour, but the researcher would also find it difficult to be in the right place and at the right time when a casual discussion of health just happened to take place. As a method of research, personal observation (participatory or otherwise) can prove to be extremely unproductive and time-wasting.

The final objection to the definition of medicine as an institution of social control is that it gives rise to an 'idealist' analysis of patients, one which exaggerates the importance of people's ideas/beliefs about health and illness and under-estimates the significance of their material and practical circumstances. People's lives are made up of work, family, friends, and neighbours, practical tasks and obligations which have to be fulfilled. All of this affects their view of their own health, the decisions they make about it and what they do when they feel unwell. None of it however is directly related to medicine or the activities of the medical profession. There are, it should also be noted, ideological forces at work in their lives other than medicine.

Having outlined these objections to the standard sociological interpretation of the relationship between medicine and society, what alternative does this study propose? The assumptions on which the analysis is based are as follows:

1. Medicine is not a unitary phenomenon; there are hierarchical and sectional differences within medicine which should be specified. Where medicine is referred to as an institution the reference is to dominant sections within the medical establishment and not to the establishment as a whole.
2. Medicine, as an institution, carries ideological weight, but the

dominance of medical ideology outside medical settings has to be regarded as problematic. Instead of assuming that medicine dominates the relationship 'ordinary people' have to health matters, the intention must be to find out whether it does, to what extent and how this has taken place. The practical basis of the relationship between medicine and society needs to be considered. Medicine is only one of a number of forces and factors that shape people's lives and their relationship to health and illness. The analysis must include an understanding of the content and quality of medical treatment available to people in specific situations as well as a knowledge of the practical constraints operating on individuals' relationships with health services.

3. Concepts and theories of all kinds are developed for use in particular social settings. The analysis of concepts of health and illness must therefore be grounded in an analysis of the practical features of specific social situations and the factors determining them. The position adopted in this study is that the people who are its subjects have responses to medicine and what it can offer them which are rational, and their understanding of what is or is not within their power to control as far as their health is concerned is realistic *from their own point of view*. They are not fatalistic, passive, or ignorant, nor are they dependent on medicine in the way some structuralists and radical accounts imply. They do however have sets of commonsense beliefs about themselves and their place in the world which affect every aspect of their lives, including how they think about health and health services.

4. The study defines its object not as 'lay concepts' but as 'commonsense ideas/theories' about health and illness. This is partly to draw attention to the fact that it is the meanings in common social currency which are being investigated, rather than individuals' ideas, and partly to avoid the opposition with professional or medical concepts that is implicit in the term 'lay'. Giddens has drawn attention to the fact that commonsense knowledge normally incorporates 'expert' and in this case 'medical' meanings:

> 'Commonsense is by no means solely practical in character – "cookery book knowledge". It is normally in some substantial degree derived from and responsive to the activities of "experts" who make the most direct contribution to the

> explicit rationalisation of culture ... Commonsense is certainly in part the accumulated wisdom of laymen; *but commonsense beliefs just as certainly reflect and embody the perspectives developed by experts.'*

(Giddens 1976: 115)

Commonsense is more appropriate to this study than the notion of lay concepts, because the idea of medicalization which it proposes as an alternative to the idea of medicine as an institution of social control (see pp. 117–23), describes a process of interaction between medical and commonsense approaches in which the medical approach is usually, but not always, dominant. Essentially, medicalization is the process through which people come to lose faith in their own knowledge and information ('the accumulated wisdom of laymen') and in their own powers of judgement. They lose it at different speeds, and in relation to different areas of expertise, but the process is defined as medicalization because the tendency is for medical rather than commonsense views to dominate.

The content of the commonsense theories with which this study is concerned may be related to a tradition of 'individualism' in East London, which in turn may be connected to the specific nature of East London labour markets. Later in the study, some connections between commonsense ideas about work and commonsense ideas about health are examined, which seem to substantiate the idea that different types of labour market, and the different ideologies associated with them, may play a part in determining the content of commonsense ideas and theories about health and illness in different social groups. For the moment we can do no more than speculate about this. In keeping with its stated aims and theoretical assumptions, the study is concerned with how the different parts of the whole way of life of the group of people who took part in it are related, and with the significance of the various parts in relation to their commonsense ideas about health and illness. We will have to wait for the study to be replicated in another part of the country with different industrial traditions and different types of labour market, before the validity of the labour market hypothesis can be properly tested.

2 Housing and the Community

Introduction

Housing, and the character of the physical and social environment are of paramount importance to people everywhere, and particularly so in East London, an area that has seen profound changes taking place at an extraordinarily rapid pace in the last fifty years. They are matters of immediate and vital concern to everyone who took part in this study. Partly for that reason, and partly in order to set the scene, it seemed appropriate to make them the focus of discussion in this, the first of the chapters dealing with the empirical material from the interviews.

There are, as it were, two levels on which the lives of the people involved in the study as 'East Enders' have to be appreciated. The first and most obvious is the material level which is concerned with the practicalities of the physical and social environment, that is, with everything from the size and composition of the local population to the numbers of local shops and public houses and the standard of work in the local authority cleansing department. There is also a second level, which is the level of ideas and stories about the place and about the people who live in it, because the East End of London has a mythological, as well as a practical, existence, and Bethnal Green, as well as being part of that myth, has a separate myth of its own.

The East End myth is a nineteenth century one of outstanding individuals – social reformers, philanthropists, moral evangelists, and the occasional criminal – set against a backdrop of poverty, squalor, and social and moral disintegration on a vast scale (Stedman Jones 1971; Williams 1973). The Bethnal Green myth is much more recent and dates only from the last war. The images with which it is most powerfully associated have their origins in the patriotic propaganda of the Home Front in the last war (Harrison 1976; Calder 1969): images of everlasting cheerfulness and co-operation, and of people working together to cope with the devastation of their streets and homes by German bombs. The myth continued after the war in the work of sociologists at the Institute of Community Studies, set up in Bethnal Green in 1954. The concept of 'community' is central to the post-war myth of Bethnal Green as the model of urban village life, a place of huge families centred around Mum, of cobbled streets and terraced cottages, open doors, children's street games, open-air markets, and always, and everlastingly, cups of tea and women gossiping together on the doorstep (Young and Willmott 1957; Young 1955; Townsend 1957; Willmott and Young 1971).

These images have been created by outsiders, observers of the East End and of the social life and mores of its inhabitants, but they have become part of what it is to live there. People who have been born and brought up in the East End almost inevitably enter into some kind of relationship with the myth – whether it is that they live it out in their own lives, that they laugh at it, reject it, feel insulted by it, take pleasure in it, or ignore it altogether.

This chapter presents the lives of the people involved in the study at both levels. It begins with a brief history of the changes that have shaped their physical and social environment over the last fifty years, and uses case histories to show their effects on local residents. The second part of the chapter examines the meaning of the concept of 'community' in two different contexts – in Young and Willmott's work at the Institute of Community Studies, and in the interviews for the present study. It attempts to show that 'community' means the same in both contexts, and that it represents a mythical ideal of social life which has more to do with morality, sentiment, and politics than it has to do with historical realities. The portrait of social life that emerges in terms of 'community' is partial and one-sided. In the sociologists' case, it is based on a selective use of evidence; and in the case of these interviews, it is based on selective recall of memories. The argument is not put forward as grounds for dismissing the notion of 'community', but for re-examining its significance, as it has been and continues to be applied to Bethnal Green.

Tower Hamlets and Bethnal Green, 1940–1980

To the outsider, the 'East End' is a vast and undifferentiated area, stretching eastwards from Aldgate on the border with the City of

London, out beyond Stratford to the middle-class suburbs of Woodford, Romford, and Ilford. To the people who live there, the 'East End', as such, does not exist, and it is the distinctive identities of Poplar, the Isle of Dogs, Stepney, Mile End, Whitechapel, Bethnal Green, and Spitalfields that count. Before 1964 these were separate administrative entities, Metropolitan Boroughs of London, each with its own town hall and local council. In 1964 they were brought together to form the much larger London Borough of Tower Hamlets, but the old loyalties remain, and to local residents it is still the old boundaries that make sense.

All the people who were interviewed in the study live in the area that used to be the Metropolitan Borough of Bethnal Green, and is now the West Bethnal Green area of the London Borough of Tower Hamlets. Tower Hamlets is a 'typical' inner city area in the sense that it has experienced very high levels of out-migration. The majority of the migrants are young, married, and economically active skilled and semi-skilled workers (Hall 1981; Howick and Key 1978; Shankland, Willmott and Jordan 1977). The people who are left in the inner city areas are often the people who have had the least choice about where to live: immigrants, single parents, unskilled workers, and the elderly (Friend and Metcalfe 1981; Cockburn 1977). They live in conditions of collective as well as individual deprivation, the relatively common experience of poverty and unemployment being made much worse by the character of the physical and social environment. In every respect – in housing, transport, shops, and leisure and public services – the standard of what is available to them is already low and is deteriorating (Syson and Young 1974; Myers 1975; Howick and Key 1978; Hall 1981).

Tower Hamlets shares the broad outlines and general features of its recent history with that of the inner city in Britain as a whole (Hall 1981), but its own particular version of that history is unique. One of the characteristics of the contemporary inner city is demographic decline (Hall 1981). In London, the population has been falling since the turn of the century; the rate of decline in the inner London Boroughs has been faster than that of London as a whole, and is accelerating, but it is fastest of all in Tower Hamlets.

One of the reasons why the decline in the population of Tower Hamlets has been so great is that it was more seriously damaged by war-time bombing than anywhere else in London. Harrison

Table 2:1   *Long-term population trends in Greater and Inner London and Tower Hamlets, 1901–1976.*

	Tower Hamlets	Inner London	Greater London
		(population in thousands)	
1901	597	4,533	6,510
1911	570	4,517	7,162
1931	489	4,393	8,110
1951	231	3,346	8,197
1961	206	3,198	7,992
1971	166	2,772	7,452
(1976)	146	2,495	7,028

(Source: Census of Population [Registrar General's estimate] Howick and Key 1978: 31)

(1976) reports 20 percent more bombs dropping in Stepney and Shoreditch than in areas ten times the size in other parts of London.

In Tower Hamlets 'overcrowding' has meant different things at different times, but, along with job losses, it has been one of the principal causes of demographic decline in the area for the past forty years. Immediately after the war, when much of the housing stock was already uninhabitable, the London County Council, in association with the local London Boroughs, initiated a programme of slum clearance. For the first twenty years, demolition proceeded at a rate of 500 units of housing per year; between 1965–72, the rate was doubled to 1,000 units (Donnison and Chapman 1965). At the same time a programme of reconstruction began in the area, and by 1971, 30,000 new housing units had been completed, more than compensating for the losses in the programme of clearances. Despite this, the period after the war was one of immense overcrowding. Thousands of people left Tower Hamlets either because they did not have enough rooms or because more than one household was occupying the same housing unit. The rate of mobility within the Borough was also unusually high, as people moved out of slum properties and into temporary accommodation before receiving their allocation to a new council property. Many of the prefabricated houses erected as temporary accommodation to cope with the overspill from the slums are still in occupation in Tower Hamlets today.

Because of the part played by local government in clearing slum

properties and rebuilding, public housing makes up a quite disproportionate share of the housing stock in Tower Hamlets. The most
recent figures (for April 1983) show that 49,000 dwellings, or 81
per cent of the housing stock, is publicly owned by the Greater
London Council and the London Borough of Tower Hamlets,
and the remaining 11,000 dwellings, or 19 per cent of the stock,
are divided between housing associations, private rented sector,
and home ownership. No accurate figures are available to show
the breakdown between rentals and home ownership, but the
approximate estimate of the Planning Department is that owner-
occupation accounts for not more than 4 per cent of the total
housing stock.

The quality of the public housing varies immensely and cannot
be described fairly in general terms. Initially the standard of
amenities, i.e. of bathrooms, toilets, access to running water, in
local authority housing was a vast improvement on slum
properties, but many local authority tenants have become increasingly unhappy and dissatisfied with the quality of their housing
over the past ten to twenty years. When the council has called
neighbourhood meetings in the Borough to find out from tenants
how they feel about their housing and about their physical environment, there have been regular and frequent complaints about
the inadequacy of playspace for children on council housing
estates; poor maintenance; slow rates of rehabilitation of older
properties; vandalism in communal areas on estates; and poor
refuse services (London Borough of Tower Hamlets: 1978).
Tenants have also regularly requested that the allocation policy
pursued by the Housing Department should take account of
where people want to live as well as of their basic housing needs.

In the past twenty years, overcrowding in Tower Hamlets has
meant residents have not had either the quality of housing or the
control over where they live, which many of them have wanted.
For many, the main reason for leaving Tower Hamlets has been
the desire to buy somewhere to live. In 1971, 41 per cent of the
families that migrated out of the Borough and 61 per cent of the
single people (making a total of 28,180 people) moved out of
rented accommodation and into owner-occupation (Howick and
Key 1978: 47).

Within Tower Hamlets, the area that was once the Metropolitan
Borough of Bethnal Green is two miles wide and three-quarters of
a mile long. Before the war, the condition of the housing stock in
Bethnal Green was unusually poor; 89 per cent of households

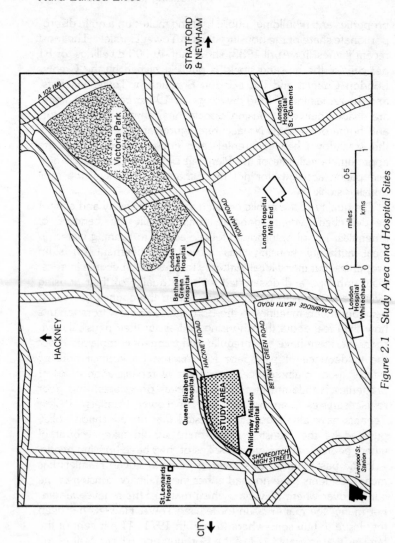

Figure 2.1 Study Area and Hospital Sites

had no bathrooms or indoor toilets, 78 per cent had no access to running water. Most people lived either in two-up, two-down terraced cottages, or in flats in the huge tenements built by private companies and charitable trusts in the nineteenth century (see Stedman Jones 1971). Housing was bad, but the area itself was not unattractive. Contemporary commentators remarked on the 'village-like atmosphere' (Glass and Frenkel 1946) in the cobbled streets where small furniture manufacturers and tailors' workshops existed side-by-side with shops, pubs, and houses. The area had an air of self-containment, cut off from neighbouring boroughs on all sides by main roads which surrounded, but did not cross it.

Bethnal Green suffered some of the worst of the bombing. It lost over 3,000 houses completely in the Blitz, and every building in the area suffered some degree of bomb damage (Donnison and Chapman 1965). In 1945, the population of Bethnal Green was less than half the size it had been at the start of the war; 48,000 rather than the 108,000 of 1931. Since the war, the programmes of slum clearance and reconstuction have radically altered the character of the place. Eliminating the mixture of land uses has been one of the principal aims. The streets of terraced cottages interspersed with factories, warehouses, and shops have been torn down and replaced by blocks of flats, massed together on large estates, surrounded by open space. Patches of under-used or derelict land and decaying buildings are a common sight, as reconstruction has not kept pace with the deterioration of building stock (LBTH: 1978).

The pattern of housing tenure in Bethnal Green is not the same as in the rest of LBTH. The proportion of public housing is smaller, 70 per cent rather than 81 per cent, and the proportion of stock owned by housing associations and private landlords is correspondingly greater. The differences are largely accounted for by the tenement buildings in Bethnal Green owned by the Guinness and Peabody Estates, and by one privately-owned estate, which will be called the 'Unicorn' Estate, which occupies a network of streets of terraced cottages in the north-west corner of the area. Eight of the households involved in the study are on this estate.

The Estate was built in the early nineteenth century by private builders who bought land leases from the Unicorn Trust. They built two-up, two-down cottages and workshops which they used themselves and rented out. The character of the Estate altered very little for almost a century and a half (the local Planning

Department describe it as 'a remnant of old Bethnal Green' (LBTH 1978), but in 1981 the Unicorn Trust sold the Estate to a private developer, since when it has rapidly begun to change. After the war the Trust, which was a charitable body, did not have the funds to do running repairs to roofs and drains, let alone the more fundamental work of repairing and rehabilitating the properties that had been damaged. Housing standards on the estate varied enormously. Some tenants installed bathrooms and indoor toilets, and sometimes even central heating, at their own expense, but others, and especially single people and old people, have not been able to afford these improvements. At a Residents' Association meeting in 1980, one tenant revealed that he did not even have electricity in the upstairs part of the house, and was using gas lights. All this is now changing. After the estate was sold, the council approved a plan to make it a Housing Action Area. As a result the properties are currently being improved with council grants to the standards of the regulations governing Housing Action Areas; indoor bathrooms and toilets, hot running water, and central heating in the downstairs part of the house are being installed throughout the estate.

The population of the estate has been extraordinarily stable over the past twenty to thirty years. Jeannie Moss and Carol McInnes have lived in the same houses for almost twenty years; Kathleen Read has been in her house almost twenty-five years, and Ben Knight has had his for thirty years. All this will now change. The new landlord's policy is to sell as much of the property on the estate as possible. Vacant houses are being sold on the open market, and existing tenants are being offered their houses at slightly less than market price. Those who can afford to, and this is usually the same people who had already done the repairs and improvements at their own expense, are taking advantage of the offer. The rest will remain as tenants until they die or move away, when their houses will be sold. The result of the changes will be to create two classes of resident on the estate – the owner-occupiers, who will tend to be married and economically active – and the tenants, who will be mostly single people and old people and some families on low incomes.

The consequences of the changes that have taken place in Tower Hamlets and Bethnal Green as a result of the war and of the programmes of slum clearance and reconstruction that followed after it have been described briefly above. Thousands of people have left the Borough since the end of the war, whilst a smaller number have moved from one temporary address to another before receiving a permanent allocation. All this has had drastic effects on the social life of local residents. Separating out the different land uses so that residential and industrial premises are not on top of each other has meant that people who are in work now travel further to work and cannot get back home at lunchtime. Formerly, members of the same family networks often lived in different households in the same street or tenement block, but their networks have been broken up, and they are separated by longer distances within the Borough and outside it. In many ways, and until recently, the Unicorn Estate represented those aspects of the past that, it appears, the present-day residents of Tower Hamlets would most like to hang on to. Although the physical standard of much of the housing on the estate was very low, the houses have gardens for children to play in. The Trust also gave priority to existing tenants in allocating new tenancies, and in contrast with the fate of families in public housing, many families on the estate have been able to stay together.

Housing case histories

The changes that have been described are reflected in the bio-graphies of the group of people that took part in the present study. Before the war, the only accommodation available to them was to rent either from private landlords or from the charitable trusts. It was not uncommon for two and sometimes more house-holds to be housed together under one roof in very restricted circumstances. This was the case for Nellie and Arthur Davies who, for the first seven years of their married lives, shared one room in Nellie's mother's house with six of their children. Cooking, washing, eating, sleeping, and sometimes working (Arthur made toy soldiers and lace doilies during his periods of unemployment to sell on the streets) all took place in the one room. Nellie's older children remember her tying them onto their chairs when she was using hot water to do the washing or cooking.

Seven people – Harold and Florrie Neagle; Ann Cullen and her daughter, Jackie Cox; Ann's sister, Betty Mayes, and her husband Daniel; and Joe Hutchinson – lived in a 'turning' which will be called Golden Row, notorious in Bethnal Green for the roughness and violence of communal life in the central courtyards of the tenements. Ann Cullen and Betty Mayes, sisters in a family of fifteen surviving children, lived in a three-roomed flat in one of the buildings. Their parents slept in the kitchen, the seven girls shared one room and the eight boys shared another across the landing where the toilet and cold tap they shared with the next door flat were situated. As the family grew up they gradually took over the flats in the building so that, when Jackie Cox was a child, the rest of the building was mostly inhabited by her aunts and uncles.

People's recollections of living in slums such as these are not rosy. Living in tenements meant not only being surrounded by filth and dirt, but it was also dark, and there was virtually no privacy. Jackie Cox is certain that the environment in Golden Row was dangerous as a playground for the children who lived there. Her mother was chronically anxious that she would catch something if she played outside with the other children, because the only place for them was the 'debris' which was infested with rats and stray cats:

> 'So consequently you was playing with rubbish and filth all the time. You just couldn't get away from it all the time. I know when I was under the Children's Hospital for a year, because I had dysentery as well. That left me with a weak stomach. I don't know whether it was just me, you know, you get these kids that are always ill, or whether, as I say, it was where we lived. 'Cause it doesn't matter how clean you were, you go to bed of a night, and you don't know who's in the toilet, because anyone could go in the toilet because the toilet was there for anyone. It was like a public toilet come to think of it.'

Jackie's uncle, Daniel Mayes, is unusual in that he left Golden Row and then came back to it when he was still young. His mother died when he was ten, and his father moved the family out to Dagenham where his sister had offered to help out. Five years later, Daniel started working in London and the combined cost of his fares and his father's fares to work on the docks was too great, and the family moved back into Bethnal Green. Daniel had loved the feeling of space in Dagenham, and the contrast between the two places allowed him to see Golden Row in a way that he vividly recalls:

> 'I'll never forget it. Because you imagine it, it was like this. You imagine coming out of Golden Row as it then was, whereby

you were living, the flats were old, the tap and sink was on the communal landing outside your street door. Your toilet was there and all. So what you had was a sort of landing with four doors, that side had a toilet but you shared a sink. In those days they were about the six-inch bell type. But people were clean, you had to be clean, but you imagine that. If you wanted a bath, you had to go to the York Hall public baths or, as a lot of people did, they bought tin baths because they couldn't afford to send their children all round the baths all the time, because it was expensive and a penny was a penny. And these baths were used. Saturday night was bath night. Well, you imagine coming from that and going to a place where you had a front and a back garden, and you went upstairs to bed. When you went into your kitchenette, which was called a scullery then, you had a nice draining board ... Not being snobbish, but as I say, you had a bathroom, you had a nice sitting room to go to and sit in the evening. And when you looked out, you looked out on flowers and lawns that you created yourself. Really and truly, to have that place, you felt different. When I was to go back to Golden Row I used to think to myself, "God, to be closed in when I was little, and now to move back". 'Cause I was older then, and understood more. Between the ages of ten and thirteen, when I went back, it was like a prison, comparing it.'

When the war came, most families with school-age children and younger were separated from each other. Kathleen Read was evacuated to the north of England, to a different town from her two younger sisters who were kept together. She did not see any cf her brothers and sisters for four years and received only occasional visits from her mother. Peggy Freeman also spent four years without having contact with any of her family; she was evacuated to Wales which was too far for her mother, who was an invalid, to be able to visit her. There were many families in which the parents either refused to allow their children to be sent away, or they fetched them back to Bethnal Green within a very short time after they had been evacuated. Betty Mayes, Ann Cullen, Joe Hutchinson, and Ben Knight were all children in Bethnal Green during the war, and normal life for them was completely disrupted. None of them attended school with any regularity and all of them moved house at least once. Betty and Ann moved three times in two years. At the end of the war none of the families involved in the study was at the same address as they had been at the beginning.

After the war, overcrowding was worse than ever, as the number of habitable properties had been so seriously diminished. The combined effects of the war, slum clearance, and a slow rate of reconstruction forced families to stay together. With one or two rare exceptions, people in every generation in the study began married life in the same house as the parents of one or other of the partners. Joan Young lived under the same roof as Nellie Davies until the eldest of her two children was nine years old:

JC: 'Were you trying to move out? Or was it all right living at your mother's?'

JY: 'It was all right. We had to take our turn like everyone else on the housing, you know. They said we was fortunate to have one room. And then when Flo [her younger sister] moved out, we got her place, so I had another room. I had a kitchen and one bedroom, which made things a lot easier. But at the same time, I still had four flights of stairs up and down to the loo, 'cause the loo was in the back garden. And I had no washing facilities up there, or anything like that. I only had a little tiny sink in the corner, just to empty water down and things like that. But me washing. I used to do me washing in buckets. Till a launderette opened down here, and I started using the launderette.'

Her remark about how lucky she was to have one room is clarified by what happened to her sister, Kathleen, when she married. At that time their eldest sister was still using the top floor room in the house for herself, her husband, and her first baby. There was literally no room in the house for Kathleen and her husband (Kathleen had been sharing a bedroom with her two younger sisters) and they could not find anywhere of their own to live. Kathleen spent the first year of married life eating her meals and spending her days in Nellie's house, and going across the road to join her husband in his mother's house in the evenings.

People who were able, reponded to overcrowding by moving out of Bethnal Green and often out of the East End altogether. In some families, the rate of out-migration has been high. Nine out of Ann Cullen's and Betty Mayes's fifteen brothers and sisters have moved out of Bethnal Green to the suburbs, to Essex and to the south coast. Ben Knight is the only one out of six in his generation to have stayed in Bethnal Green; four out of Nellie

Davies's then surviving children have moved away to the suburbs and to new towns in the home counties. Six of the Neagles's children now live in Thamesmead, Plaistow, and Dagenham. In the smaller families there are also people who have left: Carol McInnes has two brothers, one of whom lives in Essex; Joe Hutchinson's only sister-in-law lives in Dagenham. During the period the interviews were taking place, Mary Webb's eldest daughter and her husband moved out to live in their own house in Southend.

The very first phases of migration took place under council supervision. People were selected from the most overcrowded and unhealthy houses in the Borough and allocated houses on new estates, twenty miles outside London (Young and Willmott 1957: 127; Young 1955). Kathleen Read moved out of Bethnal Green under one of these schemes and was also one of the sizeable minority of emigrants who moved back in. Kathleen's first home after her marriage was two rooms above a smelting shop in a street bordering on the railway line. To reach the toilet she had to go down four flights of stairs and out through a yard full of vats of acids. The conditions were particularly damaging to her husband who had only recently been discharged after four years of treatment away from home for tuberculosis, and they were allocated a new house in Dagenham. Harry liked the house but Kathleen, who by this time had two young children, was desperately unhappy because she found living in Dagenham so depressing: 'Down at Dagenham, you didn't even hear a kiddy talking or running along, it was dead. I thought, "Let's get back to London." No, it was too quiet for me.' After two years away in Dagenham, she exchanged their house for a house in much worse condition on the Unicorn Estate, and moved back into Bethnal Green.

Slum clearance and reconstruction caused upheavals and changes for people who stayed in Bethnal Green. The local authorities' policy was to give priority to people displaced from the slums in their allocation of new tenancies, but the very fact of 'being allocated' was, in itself, unfamiliar and involved the loss of a notional degree of freedom or autonomy, not necessarily compensated for by the improved standard of housing that they were getting. Many people were sentimentally attached to their homes in the slums and felt reluctant to take up the council's offers. Nellie and Arthur Davies, and William Cox's grandfather were all evicted from terraced houses where they had lived with their entire families and moved into purpose-built flats. For the first time in their lives they had an indoor bathroom and toilet and access to hot and cold running water, but the move also meant that they lost access to a garden. The younger generations blame the move for damaging their parents' spirit and causing their health to deteriorate, and William believes that it brought forward his grandfather's death:

WC: When we moved out of the flat in Poplar, we wanted all to stay together. And they got us onto an estate in Bethnal Green. Me Mum had a ground-floor maisonette, but all they could give me Nan and Grandad was a one-bedroomed flat. He was ill when he moved into it, and from that day he really, like, I can't remember him going out of the house more than a dozen times.'
JC: 'What was wrong with him?'
WC: 'He had asthma and bronchitis, and he had cancer when he died. But for all that, when we lived in Poplar, he still got up and about. There was always something to do, like he'd go into the garden and do his flowers or see to the chickens and things like that. Although he was ill, and in and out of hospital, he would always get up and do it. When they moved him into that flat there was nothing for him to do, and he died. He'd have a bet. He used to love a bet. The nearest betting shop was like miles away, so he couldn't get down to the betting shop, so he used to lay in most of time when he was ill. He just faded away. I still, I've always said that moving him out of Poplar, that done it.'

Some were not content with their 'allocation', and when they wanted to anticipate, by-pass, or reverse an offer from the council, they organised exchanges. It was through the exchange system that many of the households in the study originally came to the Unicorn Estate, swopping council flats and maisonettes with tenants on the Estate. Carol McInnes was allocated a council flat on the seventh floor of a new block, with a balcony that she considered unsafe for her two young daughters. She swopped the flat for a house on the Estate which she saw offered in an advertisement in a local newsagent's window. Soon after, Jeannie Moss moved into a house two doors away which she swopped with the flat she had been allocated but had not as yet occupied. These were unequal exchanges in the sense that new properties were exchanged for houses in a bad state of repair and with no facilities, but both women were sure of their decision which gave them somewhere for the children to play without constant supervision.

Of the sixteen households involved in the present study, eight are on the Estate and the other eight are in council property. Mary Webb lives in a house rather than a flat, but otherwise all the council tenants are in flats or maisonettes. The quality and standard of housing in both groups – on the Estate and in council properties – is very variable. The Housing Action Area on the Unicorn Estate will introduce a uniform minimum standard, but the previous differences between the houses reflect the standards the tenants have been able to afford, and these will remain. In council tenancies the variability has less to do with individual tenants than with the basic design of the housing stock. Ann Cullen lives in a block of flats built in the nineteen-fifties. The flat itself is large, the rooms are spacious, and there is a lift service. Joan Young lives in a block built in the nineteen-sixties. The flat feels cramped, the rooms are small, and there is no lift. In both blocks the public areas are poorly maintained, the walls are covered with graffiti, and there is rubbish, and sometimes excrement and vomit on the stairs and in the corridors. Nevertheless, there is no doubt that the block of flats Ann Cullen lives in is superior. Apart from the internal design of the flats, it is a matter of where the block is situated, and of the immediate environment. Ann Cullen's flat in Bethnal Green is surrounded by grass and some trees in a quiet street where there is a mixture of different types of housing – small council houses with gardens and Victorian terraced houses. Joan Young's flat is in a block, surrounded closely by other similar blocks, next to a busy main road.

At one level, there is very little difference between being a tenant on the Unicorn Estate and being a council tenant. When it comes to making changes, being in the position of tenant means having little weight to pull. It is a position of dependence that can often leave people with a justifiable sense of their own powerlessness. Ann Cullen likes her flat, but she is frightened of the lifts and worried about being dependent on them to get help for her husband, who is in poor health. She would like to move to a ground-floor flat and to have two bedrooms (at the moment she has one) so that she and her husband could sleep separately. Her application for a transfer has the support of her GP but has not been successful, nor does she expect it to be. This is the second

37

time in her life that Ann has been in the position of having other people decide what will happen to her with regard to housing. The first time was when she waited eleven years to be moved out of her flat in Golden Row after it had been condemned by both the fire department and the health department. Her daughter, Jackie, is still angry, twenty years on:

'I daresay, if they wasn't pulled down, I daresay my Mum would probably still be there now, waiting for them to do anything about it. It's just one of the same old stories again, like, it doesn't matter who you go to. It doesn't matter if you go to the doctor's, doesn't matter if you go to the health department. They're not the ones who're affected, so they just write you down on a piece of paper and put you in an in-tray, and that's where you maybe stay for the next twenty years. So nothing ever happened, and you just got on with it. You stayed and waited.'

Council tenants who want to move now either have to put in for a transfer or organize an exchange with someone else. Joan Young has tried both. She has lived in the same flat for thirteen years, and hates it. Ideally, she would like to live in one of the new towns in the home counties her sisters have moved to, but she would be happy with anywhere away from the inner city:

JY: 'I'm not worried about having more space. All I'd like is a little house where I've got no-one underneath me, and I can walk out into a little bit of garden. It's all I want. I can't see myself getting it. No, not in this life anyway.'
JC: 'Are you not on a transfer list?'
JY: 'Oh, yes. You can wait years for that. You get shelved and forgotten.'
JC: 'How long have you been on it?'
JY: 'About two or three years. Two or three years I think it is now, it must be.'
JC: 'Is it still possible to do swops?'
JY: 'Yes. But I ask you. Who's going to swop a house for a place like this? Nobody with any sense would take a house like this.'

It is not simply a question of whether or not one can move when and where one wants. Being a tenant also means waiting on someone else to do repairs and to make improvements and alterations. When Kathleen Read first moved onto the Estate more than twenty years ago, the house she moved into needed major structural repairs to walls and foundations that had suffered bomb damage. The landlord did not do them, nor any of the repairs to roofs etc. needed since then. The council undertook to make certain alterations to her father's maisonette which would make it easier for him to get around it after he had one leg amputated. Arthur waited three weeks in hospital for the alterations to be done and was finally discharged back to the maisonette without them. The decision to make the alterations had been cancelled, after it had been made, on the grounds that they would be too costly. Arthur is now confined to the ground floor of the maisonette and is unable to use the bathroom and toilet which are on the upper floor.

Where there is a chance that their own actions will be effective, no-one in the study holds back from doing whatever is necessary. Kathleen Read's two daughters, Sharon and Joanne, were both allocated flats in other parts of Tower Hamlets, and both wanted to move back into Bethnal Green. To make sure that they were re-housed where they wanted, they toured the streets marking down vacant flats, informed the council of the addresses and of their preferences, and undertook to re-decorate the flats themselves provided they were given the allocations they wanted. Both were successful. But buying a house represents to most people their one chance of getting what they want and having control over it. Unless they can afford to buy a property, tenants on the Unicorn Estate have as much difficulty as council tenants in moving away or having the house as they want it. This explains why the offer that the new landlords have made to tenants on the Estate of buying their houses at less than market price is being taken up so quickly by those who can afford it. Not everyone who is buying necessarily wants to move away from the Estate, but they will have more choice about where they live once they are property-owners.

Although there are people in both groups of tenants who are unhappy with their housing, no-one on the Estate seems quite as unhappy as some of the council tenants. This is because they are in houses with gardens, but it is also because the previous landlords' allocation policy has enabled people to live close to their families. Many people moved onto the Estate in the old way of being 'spoken for' by relatives. A relative who was already a tenant 'spoke' to the landlord on their behalf when a tenancy on the Estate fell newly vacant, and the landlord's practice was to give priority to people 'spoken for' in this way. This was how the Chalmers and the Coxes moved onto the Estate in the nineteen-seventies, and it was the same for the Hutchinsons and the Knights over twenty years ago.

The housing case histories tell a story of poor experiences. The themes are overcrowding and squalor, chaos, disruption and the break-up of families, and the individual sense of powerlessness that comes from waiting on someone else to make the decisions about whether or not a transfer request will succeed or repairs will be done. The Unicorn Estate provides a valuable point of comparison with housing in the public sector. It is clear from the differences between the people who are residents on the Estate and the other people in the study who are council tenants, that the physical standard of housing is not all that counts. The local authority generally provides a higher standard of amenities than private rented accommodation in East London, but, in the course of time, the physical lay-out of the Estate, the fact that the houses have gardens, and the stability of the residential population have proved to be more in keeping with what local authority tenants say they would like but do not have.

The housing case histories provide a picture of the quality of material life in Bethnal Green, i.e. of the first level at which the character of the physical and social environment of the people who took part in the study should be appreciated. The case histories are the background against which the accounts of 'community', considered in the following section, should be set. At this point in the discussion, it is worth drawing attention to the stark contrast that is about to emerge between the two levels – i.e. the material and the ideological – and asking the question: is the romanticization of 'community' by the inhabitants of the community a way of making the reality tolerable?

Community

Thirty years ago, Young and Willmott's description (1957) of social life in Bethnal Green established that place as *the* model of 'community' in modern urban settings. It is not possible to do social research in Bethnal Green today without taking account of their study. By 'community' they meant two things: the existence of some kind of collective life that residents identify with, and a social life and social relationships based on reputation rather than status (i.e. on *who* people are to each other rather than *how much* they own or possess).

The definition of 'community' became stronger and more exaggerated in the course of their research careers. Originally Young defined 'community' simply as 'a sense of solidarity with other people sharing a common territory' (Young 1955: 33). In *Family and Kinship*, Young, with Willmott, began to develop the idea that 'community' is collective life, lived on the streets and in public places, but at the same time they acknowledged the central importance of privacy and of 'your home being your own' to people surrounded at very close quarters by many others:

> 'Most people have . . . had time to get to know plenty of other local inhabitants. They share the same background. The people they see when they go out for a walk are people they played with as children . . . They are the people they knew at the youth club, fellow members of a teenage gang or boxing opponents. They have the associations of a life-time in common. If they are brought up from childhood with someone, they may not necessarily like him, they certainly "know" him. If they live in the same street for long they cannot help getting to know people whom they see every day, talk to and hear about in endless conversation. Long residence by itself does something to create a sense of community with other people in the district.' (Young and Willmott 1957: 82)

By the time they wrote *Family and Class in a London Suburb* (Willmott and Young 1971), they were making the straight-forward assertion that collective life was more important than life in the home:

> 'Because they have lived in it so long, most Bethnal Greeners are surrounded by scores of people they know intimately, people who are one minute relations, another minute Borough councillors. The emphasis is not so much on the individual home, prized as this is, as on the informal collective life outside it in the extended family, the street, the pub and the open air market.' (Willmott and Young 1971: 130)

The other aspect of community, of people knowing one another because of who they are to each other rather than how much they own, relies on them having lived together and known one another a long time, but there is also something more to it. Young and Willmott saw relationships in Bethnal Green as finer, more moral and essentially *more human* than relationships on the new housing estate they called Greenleigh, because they did not involve questions of money and status:

'People in Bethnal Green are less concerned with "getting on". Naturally they want to have more money and a better education for their children. The borough belongs to the same society as the estate, one in which standards and aspirations are moving together. But the urge is less compulsive. They stand well with plenty of other people whether or not they have net curtains and a fine pram. Their credit with others does not depend so much on their "success" as on the subtleties of behaviour in their many face-to-face relationships. They have the security of belonging to a series of small and over-lapping groups and from their fellows they get the respect they need . . . In Bethnal Green it is not easy to give a man a single status because he has so many: he has in addition to the status of citizen, a low status as a scholar, high as a darts player, low as a bargainer, and high as a story teller. In Greenleigh, he has something much more nearly approaching one status because something much more nearly approaching one criterion is used: his possessions . . . People at Greenleigh want to get on in the light of these simple standards, and they are liable to be more anxious about it just because they no longer belong to small local groups. Their relationships are window to window, not face-to-face. Their need for respect is just as strong as it ever was, but instead of being able to find satisfaction in actual living relationships through the personal respect that accompanies almost any steady human interaction, they have to turn to the other kind of respect which is awarded, by some sort of strange common understanding, for the quantity and quality of possessions with which the person surrounds himself.' (Young and Willmott 1957: 134–135)

It is in the sense of their claim that relationships in Bethnal Green were morally superior to relationships in Greenleigh, that Young and Willmott can be criticized for giving a romantic and one-sided picture of Bethnal Green and of 'community' in general. One of the key characteristics they point to in Bethnal Green is that it was a 'face-to-face' community, i.e. everyone knew everyone else, if not directly then at least by repute. They emphasize the positive aspects of living in this way with other people because they regard it as a pre-condition for 'community'.

Where they acknowledge the negative aspects of 'face-to-face' living, they give them very little weight. For example, the following passage describes one of the more unpleasant aspects of life in a 'face-to-face' community, but it is positioned in a paragraph, the opening sentence of which reads, 'This exclusiveness in the home runs alongside an attitude of friendliness to other people living in the same street':

'If a person gets on bad terms with another person in the same street – like Mrs Shipway whose neighbour started "spreading stories about me and told me off for sending my children to Mum's when I go out to work" – she is also on bad terms with her family. "They're all related in this street", said Mr Lamb, "It's awful, you can't talk to anyone in the street about any of the others, but you find it's a relation. You have to be very careful." But if he is careful and keeps on good terms with his neighbours he is also on good terms with their relatives and can nod to them in the street, knowing that he will get a response. He has only to stand at his front door to find someone out of his past who is also in his present.' (Young and Willmott 1957: 85)

Young and Willmott's romantic vision of harmony and friendliness in Bethnal Green is not supported by reports of social life in 'face-to-face' communities, either in our own society in the past, or in other societies. In these studies (see for example, Roberts 1971; Bailey 1971), attention is more commonly paid to what Bailey calls the 'small politics' of everyday life which encourage enmity as much as friendship, and in which gossip and flattery, one-upmanship and ostracization are all powerful weapons. Roberts' account of his childhood in a Salford slum indicates also that people living close to poverty can have an over-riding concern with material possessions. 'The social standing of every person within the community', according to him, 'was constantly affected by material possessions, some of the slightest, and the struggle for acquisition and display of objects seemed fiercer than any known in Britain now for cars, boats or similar prestige symbols' (Roberts 1971: 17). This suggests that Young and Willmott may have been mistaken in seeing conspicous displays of ownership as a new phenomenon of the modern housing estates, and the heavily value-laden terms in which they discuss the phenomenon (the desire for money in Bethnal Green was apparently 'natural', whilst the same desire in Greenleigh was a 'compulsive urge' for things) make one suspect that they were simply more willing to acknowledge acquisitiveness in Greenleigh than to acknowledge it in Bethnal Green.

It is not novel to criticize Young and Willmott for romanticizing Bethnal Green, and it has already been said elsewhere that their description of Bethnal Green represents what they hoped to find more than what was in fact the case (Castells 1976; Deakin and Ungerson 1977). However, it is especially intriguing in the context of the present study because the interviews for the study contain public accounts of community that present a similarly romanticized version of 'community' life in Bethnal Green. These public accounts were given in answer to questions that were put to people directly about what it was like to live in Bethnal Green in the past, and what it is like to live in Bethnal Green in the present. They were statements addressed to 'the public' in the sense that they reiterated old themes that people knew were acceptable; in some instances they could be best described as extended cliches. Most of the people involved in the study identify with East London and with Bethnal Green in particular. The motivation behind the public accounts they gave of community life seemed to be to make that part of themselves that was identified with the place 'publicly' acceptable. This meant that early on in the research relationship they insisted that Bethnal Green *in the* depend so much on their "success" as on the subtleties of 'community' but that as the relationship developed, they became more critical and more revealing about the negative aspects of social life in present-day Bethnal Green and their idea of community was relegated to the past. In the same way, then that Young and Willmott compared Bethnal Green (the 'good' community) with Greenleigh (the 'bad' absence of community), people in the study compared Bethnal Green (the 'good' community) with places outside of it, or Bethnal Green *in the past* with Bethnal Green in the present. The contrast in the accounts in the interviews between the romantic memories of the past and the grim reality of the present is marked, and may have something to do with the process of memory itself. Williams (1973), for example, suggests that people want to romanticize that period of their lives that they associate with their childhood in order to conjure up for themselves the feeling of well-being that such memories often evoke.

The interviews also contain private accounts of life in Bethnal Green, and these often figured in the detail of stories about events and incidents whose ostensible subjects were not necessarily concerned with the character of social life in Bethnal Green. The private accounts often contradict the public accounts and give credence to Roberts's much more sceptical view of social relationships in 'face-to-face' communities.

Neighbourliness, friendliness, and concern for others (in the past), in contrast with selfishness, competitiveness, and snobbery (in the present), were the main themes of the public accounts of community. This was Kathleen and her sister, Joan, reminiscing about the 'turning' where they lived as children, in a two-roomed flat, with their parents and four brothers and sisters:

> KR: 'In that little turning I think we was all in the same boat. No-one had any different and no-one had any more. The doors was all open. They were only little houses such as this, but you never found a door shut against you, you know. And, as I say, we was all brought up to call them all aunts and uncles. You mustn't call them Mrs This, or Mrs That.'

> JY: 'If anyone was ill, or if anyone was in distress or anything like that, you'd see the women going in and out there. Doing things. If a woman was incapable of looking after her children, they'd go and take her washing and get it done, get the shopping and feed the kids. It was a different atmosphere than what it is now. Now all people seem to worry about is money. And what the Jones's have got, you know. But we was all tarred with the same brush, no-one had much down there, but they was a good crowd. A real good crowd.'

Daniel Mayes and Ann Cullen, sister and brother-in-law, both of whom lived as children and as adults in Golden Row, remembered life in the tenements there in exactly the same way:

> DM: 'They cleared it up after the bombing, but I know it's a shame what they did, what did happen. They parted a lot of friends. Neighbours were neighbours, they didn't come to see what you got, they came to help you. And when we all split up, there used to be a couple of local pubs and people used to meet for a bit of entertainment. You made your own. All that's gone by the board now. That's the difference that I see in Bethnal Green, in so much as the homes are better, much better to live in, but the friendliness, You've got neighbours today and they are neighbours. Years ago you had neighbours and friends, this was the difference.'

> AC: 'You get back years, you go to anybody in an old type of

flats, there's not many of them around now, they've fallen down, but there used to be your water tap and your toilets, out on the landing. Now you've all got to go out to the toilet, you've all got to go out to the tap, and this way you're seeing your next-door neighbour and you talk to them. And in the summer time we all used to stand out on the balcony and have a good laugh, but you don't here. I ain't got no balcony to go out and stand out on for a start. I don't see no-one. Even in the summer time you can come in but you don't see no-one.'

The dominant elements in the public accounts of community, as these passages from the interviews show, were the fact of *similarity* between people and the shared experience of poverty or near-poverty. Again and again people said that money had introduced a new materialism and had undermined the trust in others that provided the basis for the relationships they had with their neighbours:

Ann Cullen: 'I knew when I lived in Golden Row that I could walk out my front door and leave it open and no-one was going to rob me, because I was the same as them. But I couldn't do that here. Not for the people in here, but for the way the world is today, that's how I look at it. If I didn't lock my door, God knows what would've happened by the time I got home of a night. But in Golden Row I could go out and leave my door open, it didn't make no difference. I could trust the people there because they had nothing same as I had nothing. I think a lot of it, in these flats, is living up to the Jones's. I've got to have what she's got and all that business.'

Mick Chalmers: 'I just don't see any likeness at all now between the people of today and the people of ... I don't know whether it's because people don't want to mix with each other, or what. But you seem to have different grades of people, like, living in the same area. Like you might have a bloke who's got his own business lives next door to you now, who goes into the pub and he's got his friends, and they've got money and they're heavy drinkers and you're frightened to get in their company because you can't afford to drink with them. But it seemed like in our day, in Poplar, everyone was the same. You never had a bloke who owned his own business living next door to you. Anything like that. You was all kind of run-of-the-mill, near enough the same.'

Having money, they said, not only makes people mistrust one another's motives, it also gives individuals the means *to purchase* their own necessities and allows them to become less dependent on communal life. Private washing machines replaced the public laundry; private cars replaced weekends spent in the market or working on the garden; private televisions and videos replaced football and the local pub. Ben Knight considered television the worst of all because it meant people no longer bothered to talk to each other:

'People say "the bad old days, kids have got it better", but, you know, what's going to occupy their minds in the future when you give them the television every night and you sit down there? You say it gives you comfort. It gives you bad eyes. It gives you the lack of speech. Lack of communication with people. It gives you no knowledge. All you get is you turn round and "Did you see that last night?" There's nothing else they saw, they didn't see nothing else. Where, once upon a time, they might have been in their back gardens talking to one another, saying, "I saw so-and-so today". People don't converse like that nowadays. Today, a lot of it is self-preservation with people. They just don't care. My only care in my life is my grandchildren now, and I'm concerned with their future – and that is mercenary - that my wife is contented, my children are contented.'

The portrait of community life – past and present – painted in private accounts was very different. As well as the willingness to help the invalid neighbour, it included the turning of the blind eye to other people's troubles; as well as the open doors and the familiarity with others, it included the arguments, fights and brawls, particularly over children, and the petty snobberies that kept people apart from each other. Domestic violence was not uncommon, but neighbours who knew it was happening preferred not to become involved. To Joan Young, it had been a fact of life: 'When I think about it, you was just unfortunate if you happened to be married to a bloke who believed in knocking you about.' Whilst Kathleen, her sister, saw it principally as something to be ignored:

JC: 'Did you know much about each other's lives?'
KR: 'No, you might see a few of them with bruises, so you'd sort of say, "Well, they had a fight last night", but you never actually

heard nothing, although it was a tiny turning. Well, you could hear the same old boy that might have been drunk night after night, knowing that his kids could have done with some of the money that he was drinking.'

In place of the active concern for the welfare of others, the impression the private accounts of community life gave was that of the over-riding importance of looking after oneself and one's own. For some people this meant learning not to let others get the best of them, or their children, in physical fights, but for others it meant erecting barriers of social distance between themselves and others. The next three passages are all from interviews with people who lived in Golden Row, the place Daniel Mayes and Ann Cullen recalled so affectionately in the passages quoted above. The first is from a later interview with Ann Cullen; the next is her sister, Betty Mayes, describing their mother's strategy for coping with children in that environment; the last is from a conversation between Harold and Florrie Neagle about life in 'the turning':

Ann Cullen: 'They were rough and so were we, because you had to be. And if you weren't, then you would have got good hidings all the time, so you had to be as good as the others, and this is how it went on. This is how you was brought up to, "Right, if she hits you, you hit her back" and all this business. And you had to do it. So I suppose to me, it never made a lot of, I never really noticed because I was brought up there.'

Betty Mayes: 'She used to run after us and clobber us, yes, or if anyone else had a go at us in the street, she was out, rolling her sleeves up and all to go out. No-one couldn't touch us. As old as she was, no-one couldn't get a hair on our head and go like that [snaps her fingers in the air] to it, she'd chop their hands off. She used to say, "No-one touches. Only me. I'm the one who touches them and no-one else."'

(Harold Neagle had been telling stories about the fights in Golden Row between the residents and the police):

Harold Neagle: 'Copper wasn't allowed down there single-handed.'
JC: 'Why was it like that?'
HN: ''Cause they was all rough and ready.'
Florrie Neagle: 'All rough people, years ago.'
HN: 'All stick to one another.'

JC: 'Were you part of that?'
HN: 'Oh, yes. I came home one day from work and she's in the middle of the flats having a fight with two women. I went up to someone and said "What's all the bother?". He said, "It's your old woman having a fight".'
JC: 'Doesn't sound like you were all sticking together.'
FN: 'No, well it's kids.'
HN: 'It's children. If you had children, and she's another tenant in the flats, and her kids are hitting your kids, you'll go down after them.'
FN: 'You're not going to just stand there, are you?'

Joe Hutchinson was the victim of the petty snobbery that relies on the distinction the Neagles allude to between 'roughs' and 'respectables'. Joe was also brought up in Golden Row, but his parents lived outside the tenements, in a flat above a shop, and they saw themselves as a cut above the rest. Joe's father forbade him to go into the courtyards in the flats and to play with other children:

'My father would never let me go inside the buildings and play. He thought they were a load of roughs and if I went in there, he used to call me out. I had to obey then, rules and regulations. I could play anywhere else, but not in the courtyards.'

If we look only at the public accounts of community, the interviews for the study confirm Young and Willmott's view of social life in Bethnal Green thirty years ago. Since they represent 'community' as a thing of the past, it could well be argued that Young and Willmott were right to portray Bethnal Green as they did, and that it has since changed and become more like their description of Greenleigh. But the interviews also contain private accounts, and they suggest that not everything in the past was quite so rosy. They also demonstrate such radical differences in the way people experience community and in what they know about it that (and this is perhaps more important) the idea of 'a community life' existing at *any* time, in the past or in the present, seems something of a fiction. The most significant experiential differences are between men and women, but age and employment status are also important. This is compatible with findings in other studies (Stacey 1960; Littlejohn 1963; Townsend 1957; Willmott 1979; Frankenberg 1976) and is not in itself surprising, but it is particularly striking when the differences are between

49

men and women living in the same household. The next two quotations are from interviews with Mick Chalmers and his wife, Sarah:

> Mick Chalmers: 'I think the world has changed since I was a kid 'cause, I mean, I remember I used to live down a turning just like this, and I can remember when I was a kid, like in the summer we used to . . . all the street doors would be open and there'd be chairs out in the streets, and you'd walk along and talk to them. I mean you can walk down here in the daytime and you don't even see a soul. I mean I don't know who lives two doors away from me. You'd come home and me Nan would say, "Your Mum ain't in, she's out somewhere", and I'd go along and I'd walk in all the houses looking for me Mum. And, you know, all the doors were open and you'd just walk in.'

> Sarah Chalmers: 'See, what it is, with Mick it's different, but with me, I can walk outside the door, walk round the shops where it would take me five minutes to walk there and back, and I'll be out about half an hour, three-quarters of an hour. Because I bump into people that I know and talk and everything else. So I think it's more friendlier when you're in an area and you know people than when you don't know them.'

Mick and Sarah do not experience 'the community' in the same way as each other, so neither of them is capable of giving a fully rounded account of 'community'. The spaces they occupy – socially as well as geographically – are different. Sarah spends a great deal of time in places that Mick rarely visits, and she, in turn, rarely goes to the places he knows. Nowadays, the men rarely work locally, and most of their sense of community comes from the atmosphere in the local pub (if they are drinkers). Women, on the other hand, occupy a much wider range of communal spaces – the shops, the street, the school gates, their relatives' houses – and they have a much wider variety of contacts, not only with shopkeepers and other mothers, but also in the schools, pubs and blocks of flats where many of them are employed as cleaners.

It seems likely that what Young and Willmott described as community life in Bethnal Green was the public account of their day. (The public account of the present, when it is not being contrasted with the past, is much more positive than some of the revelations in private accounts would suggest.) If this is true, then it raises two questions that are related. First, why did they accept the public account? And, second, why do people, now as well as then, give it?

Raymond Williams's answer to these questions would be that the idea of community, in academic and popular discourse, allows people to express needs they feel that are produced, but not satisfied, in the way they live their lives (Williams 1973). Ideas of community, he says, express:

> 'not only in disguise and displacement but in effective mediation or in offered and sometimes effective transcendence, human interests and purposes for which there is no other immediately available vocabulary. It is not only an absence and distance of more specific terms and concepts; *it is that in country and city, physically present and substantial, the experience finds material which gives body to the thoughts.*' (Williams 1973: 291, my emphasis)

And with regard to the ideas of community promoted by Young and Willmott, and reproduced in the public accounts in the interviews for this study, he writes:

> 'It is not so much the old village or the old back-street that is significant. It is the perception and affirmation of a world in which one is not necessarily a stranger and an agent, but can be a member, a discoverer in a shared source of life.' (Williams 1973: 298)

In Williams's view, regardless of whether or not they are historically authentic, people's ideas of community offer insights into their emotional and psychological states. The research of another member of the Institute of Community Studies provides some useful clues as to why the idea of community should have been especially appealing in Bethnal Green at the time Young and Willmott were doing their empirical work, and why it should continue to be so in the present. Marris (1974) has argued that the experience of losing one's home in the demolition of slums is comparable to that of losing a close relative:

> 'The definition of a slum is also a definition of the people who live there. Their own attachment to the neighbourhood is reinforced by the insistence of authority that in moving they must change not merely their surroundings, but the way they live. A situation is created which resembles bereavement in the sudden and irretrievable nature of the loss, yet provides no

process akin to mourning by which the loss can be assimilated and the essential continuity of life restored.' (Marris 1974: 56–7)

If the need to mourn the loss of a home and a neighbourhood is not recognised, then people can, as it were, 'get stuck' at some point in their grief over the loss, and fail to assimilate and eventually overcome it. Slum clearance does not necessarily carry the same meaning for everyone involved, and Marris suggests that it may be the people who remain in the area and witness it changing out of recognition, rather than the ones who make a clean break with the past and move somewhere else, who suffer most. He describes three 'abortive' processes of bereavement, all of which result in the person changing the lost object, either by under-valuing it, or by over-valuing it, or by eradicating it from their memory altogether. One of these may help to explain the nature of those public accounts of Bethnal Green that locate 'community' as a thing of the past. This is chronic grief, in which the bereaved person refuses to let go of the past, but holds on to it and mummifies and romanticizes it instead.

In popular imagery as well as in the imagery of academic community studies, the idea of community is one of a self-regulating society which has the qualities of warmth and sympathy, generosity and mutual self-help (Bell and Newby 1972). Whatever Bethnal Green was like before the war – and it is likely to have had its share of gossip, one-upmanship, and conflicts – there is no doubt that social life there was drastically altered in the course of the war and its aftermath. Men who formerly worked around the corner and returned home for their midday meal, so that they were around all day, had further to go to work and stayed away all day. Families that formerly shared the same table, even though they lived in separate households, were now spread out all over the Borough and often much further afield. When Young and Willmott did their research in Bethnal Green in the 'fifties, the pre-war pattern of social life was already disappearing, and it is arguable that the urban village community they described, and that local residents presented to them, was an image that was gaining in significance precisely because of the threat of the rapid social changes already underway. (Castells makes a similar criticism of a French study of a city area in the process of renewal in which, in a comparable situation, the authors of the study accepted the local residents' 'mythical and over-harmonious image of community' (Castells 1976: 58).) In other words, the public account of community Young and Willmott were given, and which they accepted, and which is still given today, is an image of a way of life that people want but do not possess.

Marris's theory that the mourning process is as relevant to being evicted from a slum as it is to experiencing the death of a close relative, and that in both cases it has to be completed if the person is to be able to let go of the lost object and adapt successfully to change, helps to explain the emotional dynamic underlying the significance of public accounts of community *for the individual*, and may also explain the considerable success that ideologists of the right have had with their use of the notion of 'community' in East London. In this particular political rhetoric, the concept of community, with its associations with the ideal of sameness between people, which is also a hostility towards anything that is new or different, has underpinned the growth of support for parties of the far right whose chief political platform is racism. This is a different negative aspect of community from those that have been previously mentioned. It is not the negativity that arises out of 'face-to-face' living in too close proximity, but another, darker side of that 'sense of solidarity' that Young and Willmott have not been alone in promoting as central to the notion of community. Marris's theory of what happens when the process of bereavement is abortive may also explain some of the conservatism and the hostility towards change that finds expression in political support for the National Front. There is a strong sense of community in Bethnal Green, but it should be noted that where there is belonging, there is also not belonging, and where there is in-clusion, there is also ex-clusion. In East London, the dark side of community is apparent in a dislike of what is different, which finds its clearest (but by no means its sole) outlet in racial prejudice. With one or two exceptions, everyone involved in the present study expressed some degree of hostility towards the local population of Bengalis, and towards West Indians and Asians more generally. Significantly, their main objection is to racial groups whom they see as more interested in maintaining a separate cultural identity than in becoming more 'like us'. At heart, it seems, the real ideological significance of the idea of community in present-day East London lies in its opposition to everything that is new and different and to the possibility of change.

Conclusion

This chapter has been mainly concerned with issues of housing and the community, and it has used them to develop the theme of difference between public and private accounts introduced in the previous chapter and taken further in the chapters to follow. There are two features of this discussion that recur in later chapters and are particularly significant for the analysis of the relationship that people involved in the study have to matters connected with their health and with the health service. These are: first, the observation that social scientists – 'experts' of a kind – have played a part in creating and sustaining public accounts (in this case public accounts of 'community'); and, second, that public accounts, though integrally connected to people's experience, are only *partial* reflections of that experience.

3 Work

In order to know the people involved in this study, it is necessary to understand their relationship to work (for women, this includes domestic work and childcare) and to the family. They perceive both aspects of life as crucial in the construction of a person's identity. For men, it is accepted that work is the more important of the two; for women, it is their position in the family and at home. Together, these two aspects of life constitute what they define as 'normal', meaning both 'that which is common and usual' and 'that which ought to be/is to be expected'.

In the context of a study concerned with the relationship of individuals to health matters, definitions of 'normality' have a special significance. One of the most basic ways in which people define illness is as an occurrence that disrupts 'normality' and is itself 'abnormal'. Again, a double meaning is implied; illness is 'abnormal' in the sense that it is 'not what ought to be/is not to be expected'. If we can understand the broader meaning of 'normality' for the people who were interviewed, we are more likely to understand the definition of 'abnormality' they apply in cases of illness.

This chapter is concerned with work, the next with family life. The discussion of work precedes that of family life for two reasons. First, it includes a brief economic history of Tower Hamlets over the past fifty years, which supplements the history of housing and population changes in the previous chapter and fills out the background to the interviews with individuals and families in Bethnal Green. Second, the discussion of sexual segregation in the East London labour market (which is more extreme than in labour markets nationally) will help to clarify the economic background to the domestic and family relationships examined in the next chapter.

The material in Chapters 3 and 4 introduces the people who took part in the study more fully than they have been introduced already and attempts to provide the understanding of the way that the different parts of their lives are integrated into the whole, anticipated in Chapter 1. The two chapters are also meant to be read as part of a wider argument about the relationship that these people have to health and illness and to the health service. Both chapters are especially concerned with the moral attitudes that are brought to bear on the subjects of work and of family life, and subsequent chapters show that the same attitudes inform people's approach to matters of health generally. The argument running through the separate chapters is that each aspect of people's lives needs to be understood both on its own and in relation to all the other aspects. The interpretation of commonsense ideas and theories about work and about employment should not be separated from the meanings associated with family/domestic responsibility.

The chapter begins with an outline of the economic history of Tower Hamlets, the purpose of which is to demonstrate the extent to which the present-day residents of Tower Hamlets are dependent on an ailing and restricted labour market in which it has become increasingly difficult for men and women to find jobs. This is followed by brief occupational histories of the men and women involved in the study, illustrating the effects the local labour market has on the lives of individual residents in Tower Hamlets and giving some idea of the nature of the experience on which the discussions about work that took place in the interviews were based. The main part of the chapter is devoted to description and analysis of the structures of moral belief that underlie attitudes towards work and the accounts of work – both public and private – contained in the interviews. Briefly, people in the study take it for granted that both men and women are obliged to work, whether inside or outside the home, and they also believe that people demonstrate their worth in the way that they respond to that obligation. Basically, people who accept it are considered to be 'good', meaning responsible and worthy of respect, whilst people who deny the obligation to work or who try to find a way out of it are considered to be 'bad', meaning irresponsible and discreditable. These are simplifications, and the content of the moral beliefs that are applied to work is in fact more complicated and contains assumptions about the position of the individual person in relation to work that are contradictory. The analysis of public and private accounts of work presented in the chapter shows that people find different ways of making sense of work, all of which amount to the same thing – an acceptance of what is conventionally understood as 'the capitalist work ethic'. In public accounts they put forward the positive aspects of work and the positive reasons for doing it. In private accounts they tend to be more concerned with the content of the work and of the employment relationship and with the ways they had found of making their experience of work tolerable.

The labour market in Tower Hamlets: 1930–80

The East London economy has been in decline since the last quarter of the nineteenth century. Before the past war, Tower Hamlets had two main employers: the docks, along with the transport and distribution industries attached to them, and small manufacturing firms producing goods mainly for personal consumption such as boots and shoes, furniture, clothes and food and drink. The area divided into geographically specific labour markets: men in the boroughs closest to the river were employed in the docks, whilst men living in the boroughs closer to the City and the West End, including Bethnal Green, were either small manufacturers or their employees. The small firms were under threat from factory-based producers in other parts of the country; by the time the war started, the boot and shoe industry had collapsed, and the furniture industry was struggling to survive the competition. In contrast with other areas of London such as the Great North and Great West Roads where new electrical and light engineering industries were developing, no new industries were introduced into the East End to replace those that were disappearing.

The war accelerated the rate of industrial decline in Tower Hamlets. Once it was over, the local economy was far more concentrated and specialized than was typical of inner London. By the nineteen-fifties, 60 per cent of employment in Tower Hamlets was in three industries – furniture, clothing, and food and drink; the rest was largely accounted for by the docks. Employment was decreasing, although this did not become apparent immediately because large numbers of people were moving out of the area, and for a while it was not difficult for people who remained in the borough to find jobs. Young and

Willmott who were doing research and living in Bethnal Green at the time, described the local economy as stable and buoyant and foresaw no employment difficulties in the future for men who stayed in the borough (Young and Willmott 1957).

In the nineteen-sixties, the impact of the changes that were taking place was more apparent. Migration out of the borough continued but at a slower and steadier pace, and it became obvious that opportunities for employment in the borough were decreasing. At the same time it was becoming clear that what was happening in Tower Hamlets was not unusual or unique. The inner areas of all the large cities in Britain were losing jobs. Manufacturers were under pressure to cut costs and reorganize production and were moving away from inner city premises that were often too old and too small to rationalize effectively (Hall 1981; Dennis 1978). In the ten years 1961–71, London as a whole lost 24 per cent of jobs in manufacturing, and the inner London boroughs lost an even greater proportion, 31 per cent (Howick and Key 1978). Almost 400,000 manufacturing jobs in London disappeared between 1966 and 1974; 44 per cent were in firms that went bankrupt or closed down and were not replaced by new firms, while 27 per cent were in firms that moved to premises outside London, or relocated parts or the whole of their London base to existing subsidiaries elsewhere in Britain (Dennis 1978). The boroughs that were affected the most were those in North and East London. Tower Hamlets suffered the worst job losses of all, closely followed by its immediate and close neighbours, Islington, Hackney, and Newham. Table 3:1 shows the impact on employment in these boroughs and in Newham and Barking:

Table 3:1   *Unemployment rates for selected boroughs, 1961 and 1971*

Borough	1961		1971	
	Male	*Female*	*Male*	*Female*
Tower Hamlets	2.6	1.0	6.2	3.4
Hackney	2.2	1.3	4.8	4.0
Newham	1.6	1.3	4.9	3.9
Islington	2.6	1.5	5.2	4.1
Barking	1.1	1.3	4.0	3.3

(Source: Census 1961, 1971; London Borough of Tower Hamlets 1978: 37)

The exceptionally high rate of job losses in Tower Hamlets was due to the closure of the docks rather than to a decline in manufacturing. Apart from the dockers themselves, workers in the transport and distribution industries connected to the docks also lost their jobs. Between 1961 and 1971, 26,000 men were put out of work, of which the majority (18,120) were lorry drivers, packers and warehousemen (Howick and Key 1978: 10). For a short time, manufacturing in Tower Hamlets survived the financial pressures generally operating on manufacturing industry because it was, as it always had been, based in sweat shops. Employers in Tower Hamlets were already managing to keep overheads down, not by modernizing production and making it more efficient, but by cutting costs, renting poorly maintained premises, supplying the workers with inadequate heating, using outmoded and secondhand machinery and, especially, employing cheap (i.e. female and immigrant) labour. The units of production were often small enough to avoid inspection by the Health and Safety Executive. In 1974, for example, 70 per cent of the places of employment in Tower Hamlets employed less than ten people, and 97 per cent employed less than fifty (London Borough of Tower Hamlets 1978: 32). The industries that suffered in Tower Hamlets in the nineteen-sixties were industries employing men, especially skilled men (LBTH 1978: 17). Between 1961 and 1971, male employment in Tower Hamlets decreased by 25 per cent, compared to a decline of 17 per cent in female employment for the same period. Female employment was less affected because of the high proportion of women working in the clothing industry (i.e. sweat shop production). Over 20 per cent of women who worked in Tower Hamlets, and over 50 per cent of the women working in manufacturing, were employed in the clothing industry (Howick and Key 1978: 12).

In the past ten years, Tower Hamlets has continued to record the highest rates of unemployment in London. It has lost jobs at approximately twice the rate of other Inner London boroughs, and three times the rate of the Greater London boroughs. Figures for the first half of the decade show changes in the pattern of job losses in Tower Hamlets (see *Table 3:2*). The loss of jobs in transport and distribution has slowed down now that the closure of the docks is finally over, but losses in manufacturing have increased and have not, as they have in some areas, been offset by the development of the new, so-called 'growth industries', i.e. professional, banking, finance, and scientific services. As a result, it has

Table 3:2   *Employment by Industry Group, Tower Hamlets and Greater London, 1971 and 1975*

Industry Group	Tower Hamlets			Greater London
	1971 (000)	1975 (000)	% change	% change
Manufacturing	32.7	23.3	− 29	− 14
Growth services	25.8	25.8	0	10
Other industries	40.0	34.5	− 14	− 3
Total	98.5	83.6	− 15	− 4

(Source: Dept of Employment data for Poplar and Stepney Local Employment. GLC based on DE data for Greater London (Howick and Key 1978: 14))

been women and unskilled workers, who had previously survived job losses in the local area, who have begun to be affected (Howick and Key 1978).

Commuter flows in and out of the borough show that the people most affected by job losses in Tower Hamlets have been local residents. Most people who work outside the borough work in the immediate surrounding boroughs where unemployment is almost as high as it is in Tower Hamlets. (The most recent figures for unemployment in three boroughs – Tower Hamlets, Hackney, and Islington, in the autumn of 1983 – show rates of 20, 15, and 18 percent, respectively.) There has been some decline in the numbers leaving Tower Hamlets to work outside the borough, but it is not as steep as the decline in numbers working locally. The groups most affected by the recent job losses have been semi – and un-skilled male workers, and women.

The changes that have occurred in the Tower Hamlets labour market over the last fifty years have thus been uneven and often out of step with those elsewhere in London and nationally. In comparison with other parts of London, there has been a striking lack of new initiatives in the East End. For Tower Hamlets residents the opportunities for employment have decreased rapidly. Twenty years ago men were more seriously affected than women because of the loss of jobs in the docks and the industries related to it; women's jobs in sweatshop-based manufacturing seemed relatively secure. In the last ten to fifteen years, however, manufacturers have closed down and moved out of the area and women's opportunities for work locally have also diminished.

Occupational histories

The occupational histories of the men and women who were involved in this study, and of other members of their families, are an indication of the ways in which the developments in the local economy outlined above affect the residents of Tower Hamlets.

The great-grandfathers in the study families, i.e., the men who were old enough to have fought in the First War, represent a cross-section of typical East London occupations. Three of them drove lorries; two were scrap dealers and market salesmen; amongst the rest was a docker, a barge-builder, a precision engineer, a furniture-maker and french polisher, and a local authority manual worker.

The working experience of the nine men who were actually interviewed is wide and varied, but it is largely concentrated in trades and industries traditionally associated with East London. The eldest amongst them – Ben Knight and Daniel Mayes – are, respectively, a market trader and a security man with a City bank. Both men left school at the age of fourteen and began apprenticeships which were then interrupted by the war. After the war, Ben Knight worked for two years as a bus driver with London Transport before becoming a porter at Billingsgate Market. Porters, the men who unload the lorries and set out the displays, are the lowest paid workers in the market. But having managed to get into the market, Ben rapidly became first a salesman and eventually a partner in the firm that employed him. Daniel Mayes became a wood machinist after the war. He worked in a wood mill for a short time before joining a firm reproducing antique furniture.

He remained with the same firm for twenty-eight years, and was promoted to the position of being in charge of the shop floor, with responsibility for two workshops and about twenty men under him. In 1978, when Daniel was fifty-eight, the firm closed and he was made redundant. Almost immediately, he succeeded in finding work as a doorman in the City, a post he still held two years later when he was interviewed.

Joe Hutchinson and Stan Flowers are a few years younger than Ben and Daniel, the important difference between them being that the two younger men were still at school during the war. Both of them left school at fourteen without qualifications, their last few years at school having been very seriously disrupted by the wartime bombing in East London. Joe Hutchinson delivered milk until he was sixteen, when he joined a firm of importers working in the docks, and became delivery boy, then lorry driver and, eventually, transport manager. In 1969, after he had been with the company for twenty-two years, it moved to premises outside London, and Joe was made redundant. He spent a year on the dole before taking up his present job with another firm of importers where he controls the stock. Stan Flowers joined the sawmill where he had previously been part-time tea-boy when he left school, and remained in wood-machining and furniture-making until his death at the age of fifty-nine in 1980. He was never formally trained as a wood-worker, and spent his life moving between a number of different firms locally, depending on the availability of work and the distances involved in travelling to work. He was on short-time, working three days a week, before he was taken ill. He had been with his current employers for three years.

Mick Chalmers is nearly forty. He left school at fifteen without qualifications and has since begun various apprenticeships – in boiler-making, pewter-making, and at sea – without completing any of them. In the past twenty-odd years he has had semi-skilled jobs in factories and worked as a labourer. Prior to his current job as a drayman with one of the local breweries in Tower Hamlets, he worked for an engineering firm, assembling missile components.

William Cox is the only one of the men to have completed an apprenticeship and secured a qualification (as an electrician). He worked for three years as an electrician outside London in the nineteen-seventies but found that there was not enough work and, after working as a builder's labourer for a short while, he moved back to London and joined his uncle's haulage firm as a lorry driver. Recently his uncle's health has been failing and William has taken on much of the responsibility for the firm; he expects to become a partner before long.

The youngest man in the study is Andy Mayes. He is twenty-three and a medical student. He is the only one of the men who stayed at school beyond the minimum leaving age, and the only person in the study who has continued in full-time education since leaving school.

The pattern of the women's working lives is different from that of the men. It is determined as much by their passage through the life-cycle in the context of a traditional sexual division of labour, in which they are responsible for running the household and looking after the children, as by the state of the local economy. The eldest women who were interviewed – Nellie Davies and Florrie Neagle – did unskilled work in factories (packing) until they married, but after they had children they did not go back to work outside the home. The other, younger women all worked up to their first pregnancy and their subsequent employment has been dictated by the requirements and responsibilities of their domestic position. Their working lives vary according to how old they are, how many children they have, the age of the children, and the age difference between the children. For those who are still married (as opposed to widowed or divorced), the adequacy of their husband's earnings in relation to household expenditure is also a factor in whether they have outside jobs and how much time they spend working outside the home.

The middle-aged women who were interviewed all left school at the minimum leaving age. The ones with qualifications and school leaving certificates do secretarial work and clerical work in offices; the ones without qualifications are either cleaners or shop assistants, or they do semi-skilled manual work in local sweat-shops. Ann Cullen, for example, is a machinist in the clothing industry. She is the only one of the women who has worked without interruption since she left school. She stopped working for six weeks when her daughter was born, but went back to work immediately, leaving the baby with her sister. When she had the child her husband was working for the local council and was poorly paid. He subsequently became a scrap dealer and then began to run stalls selling clothes in street markets. His income is more than adequate to provide for him and Ann, but she continues to work now out of choice. The other women in her generation who were interviewed stopped work when they had their first child and usually went back to work once the children were in school. In Mary Webb's case, this has meant going back to work in the past five years; she has eight children between the ages of twenty-five and ten and for the previous twenty years she had been at home looking after them. Mary's sisters, Kathleen and Joan, have worked on and off since their children were born, in part-time jobs as office cleaners and factory workers.

The pattern of the women's working lives in the younger generation is much the same. Joanne Goode and Sarah Chalmers left school without qualifications and have had a variety of factory and cleaning jobs. Joanne's sister, Sharon, and Jackie Cox, on the other hand, both managed to get secretarial qualifications while they were still at school, and they have had jobs in local offices and banks. When they were interviewed, Sarah and Sharon were working part-time, Sarah as a machinist and Sharon as a cashier in a City bank. Joanne and Jackie were technically unemployed and at home looking after young children. In fact, Joanne had an evening cleaning job and did seasonal outdoor work at home making soft toys, when the work was available, and Jackie did the paper work for her husband's business at home, in the evenings.

On the whole, the men and women involved in the study have exercized very little choice in the matter of work. The choices they have made have largely been negative, such as the choice Ben Knight and Mick Chalmers made not to work with their fathers, or Stan Flowers's choice not to take work that would mean travelling long distances. For the men as well as for the women, the fact of early marriage and youthful parenthood, often before or by the time they were in their early twenties, is a factor that has determined the kind of work they do. Ben Knight joined London Transport when he left the Army because the company had a reputation for paying well and he had a wife and two children to support; Mick Chalmers gave up an apprenticeship to become a labourer in order to earn enough to support a wife and child at the age of nineteen; William Cox gave up working as an electrician when he found himself unable to earn enough to support his family; he, too, became a labourer. For most of the women, having a child has meant leaving work and staying at home, and subsequently having very little choice over the nature of their paid employment outside the home. The women take whatever work is available and compatible with their domestic responsibilities at the time that they need it.

In the occupational histories of the men, two factors are particularly significant in relation to the type of work they do. One is their level of education/qualification when they leave school; the other is the nature of their personal contacts. With the exception of Andy Mayes who stayed at school and went into the sixth form (along with two other people in the school), all the men left school without qualifications. Ben Knight's and Daniel Mayes's education continued whilst they were in the services during the war. Ben described himself as 'hardly able to read and write' when he left school, but he learned to do both in the Air Force and believes that without that he would not have become the successful businessman he is now:

'I was terrible. My results, I was good at religious, at English, my writing was terrible. I used to get Fair, Fair, Fair, but nothing Excellent and nothing Very Good. Arithmetic, I was shocking at Arithmetic. But I think the forces, it made me study a bit. I studied and I learned to write properly, and my writing now is pretty fluent. People tell me that I've got my father's hand a little bit now, the flow. But there, as I say, I think the services done me a world of good.'

Daniel Mayes received a basic training in woodwork in the Army, and on the strength of it rose to become the head of the mill in a firm reproducing antiques. In contrast, Joe Hutchinson and Stan Flowers both left school without qualifications and received no further education or training at any point in their lives. Both men talked of their awkwardness and lack of confidence in applying for jobs, when they were interviewed. Joe described himself as doubly handicapped by his lack of formal qualifications and his difficulties in knowing how to put himself forward to potential employers, especially on paper:

'Once you're off the ground you're all right, but I think once you go, it's just butterflies and you withdraw, because you don't know what type of people they are that you'll be up against and what they'll want to know. This is what, in modern society, you seem to draw back where people are possibly far more educated than yourself who are interviewing you and they know what it's all about. And they don't know your capabilities and you can't explain your capabilities to them. A variety of form filling and, let's be quite honest, most forms or interview forms now want to know what "O" levels or CSEs you've had, and once I put down my education there's nothing like that 'cause they weren't there in them days. So I have to say and just put down nothing for all this schooling, No, No, No to all these variety of things, and immediately you think by filling in them forms you won't stand a chance. I think that is the biggest drawback in this modern age. So you're back to "better the devil you know than the devil you don't know".'

Of all the men, the ones who have done the best for themselves are the ones who have had special or privileged contacts, and who have used them to become self-employed. The two men in question are Ben Knight and William Cox. In Ben's day it was not possible to work in Billingsgate without being 'spoken for'; Ben had personal contacts in the market and he used them to get into the market where he worked himself up to the top of the firm that originally employed him. William Cox will not have to work as a manual worker and lorry driver for the rest of his life because, through his uncle, he will eventually be running his own business. Neither Ben nor William can guarantee what their earnings will be, but they are in control over whether or not they have a job to go to. By comparison, the other men have very little control over their working lives. Stan Flowers in the furniture industry was accustomed to being laid off and put on part-week working all his working life. Daniel Mayes and Joe Hutchinson were made redundant after working for the same employer for twenty-eight years and twenty-one years, respectively. Neither qualifications nor experience, nor length of service gave these two men control over the fundamental issue of whether or not they had a job to go to.

The moral significance of work

So far, the picture presented in this chapter is one of a local economy in decline and offering a restricted and diminishing range of job opportunities to people who live in Tower Hamlets. The occupational histories of the people who took part in the study illustrate what this means to individuals who want, as most people do, to work locally. Their chances of finding work at all are worse than anywhere else in London, and their options are limited to semi- and un-skilled manual work in a small number of industries and service occupations. Some of them succeed in finding different kinds of work and work that will take them out of the local labour market, but they are people who have the right contacts or people who leave school with qualifications. They are the exceptions. Most people who are brought up and educated in Tower Hamlets do not have the resources, personal or otherwise, that would allow them to move away from the constraints imposed by the state of the local labour market.

When they talked about work in their interviews, most people hardly mentioned the state of the local, or for that matter the national, economy as something that determines their relationship to work and to employment. Most the time they discussed employment in individual terms, i.e., as the product of individual effort and a sign of the person's sense of responsibility. It would be wrong to suggest that there was absolutely no discussion at all of national or local economic developments or of the ways in which they were personally affected by them. Some people did talk about the recession and rising unemployment: William Cox, for example, attributed his difficulties in finding work as an electrician to the slump in the building industry; Stan Flowers said that falling demand was the cause of short-time work in the furniture-making industry, and Mick Chalmers was expecting to be made redundant by the brewery because of falling demand and rising costs in the industry. Nevertheless, the framework within which people chose to talk about work in the interviews was one of morals. They continually associated work with meanings that are 'moral', in the sense that they were posed as answers to general philosophical questions about the nature of individuals' responsibility for themselves and for what happens in their lives, and as the basis for assigning categories of 'good' and 'bad' to individual behaviour.

The public accounts of work in the interviews put forward two separate and contradictory but neverthless connected arguments about the position of individuals in relation to employment. Often the same person espoused both arguments in the course of one interview, so that clearly, at the level of everyday reasoning, it was either not apparent that the arguments were contradictory, or they were made to seem compatible.

The first argument explains the position of the individual in relation to work as part of a 'natural order of things', and can be expressed as the idea that 'you are what you are meant to be'. People are naturally suited to different kinds of work, and most people do the work that naturally suits them. 'Natural suitability' or 'fitness' for work is partly a matter of one's sex – men do men's work, women do women's work – and partly a matter of what is vaguely conceived as 'natural abilities', but is most commonly seen as 'fitness' of intellect. The more intelligent you are, the more likely it is that you will have a 'difficult' job that will be well rewarded financially and in terms of status. This argument exonerates individuals from responsibility, or credit, or blame, for their occupational position. It is understood that occupational inequalities are merely the reflection of 'natural' differences that exist between people, with respect to their 'natural' abilities/intellect. Ann Cullen, for example, has been a machinist all her life, but she regards her daughter, Jackie, as more intelligent than herself, and accepts it as 'right' and 'natural' that Jackie should do secretarial work which is more highly paid and more prestigious than machining:

> 'If you've got it, you've got it, if you ain't, you ain't. That's how I look at it, but it's never bothered me because I've always earned a living.'
>
> 'Whether you're a woman or not, whether you're married and have got chidren, you have to stay home for a certain time, when your children grow up and you have to go back to work, to be educated is a very good thing. I know that my Jackie hasn't got to sit at a machine like I do and slog her guts out for nothing like I do. My Jackie could go and get a good job. I know she's got babies, but when the little one goes to school, she's still a young person to go and get an office job. She's going to get good money for the work that she does, she hasn't got to go and sit in a factory like I do.'

Psychologically, the idea that the occupational hierarchy reflects natural, qualitative differences between individuals, encourages people to accept their place in the social hierarchy, but it is also one of the mainsprings of English snobbery. The idea was generally accepted by most people involved in the study, but whether or not they *liked* the idea was a different matter. Daniel Mayes has a positive view of social and occupational hierarchies: he describes the senior personnel of the bank where he is employed as a doorman as 'toffs' and 'gentlemen' and says that he respects them for 'having made it'. It is not difficult to see why this should be the case. Daniel himself was a skilled worker for most of his working life, one up from his father who was a docker. Daniel's son is training to become a doctor, and will one day be one of those rare individuals who do indeed 'make it'. Daniel and his wife are acutely aware of their son's actual and potential success and its social significance:

> 'I always say that you treat people as they are. In three years' time, touch wood, my kid, to me, will be a little bit higher than me. Because he is a professional man so therefore he's got to be that little bit higher, ain't he? I mean now he comes in here and talks normal, but in three years' time he will be that little bit above.'

Mick Chalmers's understanding of social and occupational hierarchies is less sympathetic than Daniel's. Mick is a manual worker, and as a manual worker he feels looked down on by office workers and people who have their own businesses:

'I think a lot of people, if they've got a bloody good job and they're high up, they seem to look down on you. "What sort of job do you do?" "I sweep the roads. What do you do?" "I'm er, got me own business like. I've got people working under me." You know what I mean? And straight away you're gone, wallop. You feel it's just like going to work. I'm talking to a bloody governor like.'

The element of fatedness in the idea that 'you are what you are meant to be' carries a sense of moral as well as natural fitness, and is quite at odds with the second argument about individuals in relation to work, which is that 'life is what you make it'. It is this argument that carries the full weight of moral meanings with which work is associated and that underlies the judgments people make about each other, based on their reputations as workers. People who are 'good', take responsibility for themselves and for others in their families, they earn their way and they work hard for their living; people who are 'bad' are people who are lazy, who expect to get something for nothing, who scrounge and do not have a job to go to. The nature of a person's job is irrelevant; they can be a plumber, an engineer, a manual labourer, a doctor, or a housekeeper. What matters is the spirit with which they go about their work and the energy they put into it. People are not condemned for being at the bottom of the occupational hierarchy, but they are condemned if they do not appear to be trying to work hard and if they seem to be 'wasting their talents'. For example, Sarah Chalmers' sister had the opportunity to 'better herself' by going to the local grammar school but she did not take it, something for which Sarah has very little sympathy:

'My sister, she should have gone to grammar school and gone further but she wouldn't go 'cause her mates never went. Now my sister, I think she wasted what talent she did have where she should have gone ahead. Because when she left school she ended up as a upholstery slipper. Sewing the bloody cushions. She wasted it.'

Notions of 'making the most of oneself' and of thereby 'deserving' what one gets, connected to the argument that the occupational hierarchy is in keeping with a 'natural order of things', produce a non-contradictory, moralistic synthesis in which the hierarchy is an act of nature but it is up to individuals to put effort into achieving their rightful place within it. Each person's duty, therefore, is to make the most of their 'natural abilities':

> Ann Cullen: 'When you grow up and you're at fifteen and sixteen, then your life is what you make of it, not what other people do, it's what you make it. If you want to go out and be whatever with brains, I know you can't buy brains, if it's not there, there's nothing much you can do about it. But there again, even if you haven't got any brains you can still say, "I'm going to do a machining job or such a job". My nephew, he's a doctor of science and that boy only lived down here, he only went to ordinary junior school. It's only what he wanted to be and he worked at it and he worked hard.'

Mick Chalmers's understanding of the importance of education to his daughter expresses the balance that parents try to achieve between the two arguments:

> 'Years ago, it didn't matter with a girl because nine times out of ten they got married anyway and did not go to work. But as things are now, women are going to work, so I think it is important that the girl, I mean if she's got to have to go to work I'd like to think she could go and do a little office job where she could get dressed up and go and sit down and walk out of there clean and everything than have to go to, say Lesney's, the toy factory, earning peanuts watching little dinky toys going by and putting rubber wheels on the bloody things. To me, I don't blame a kid if it's not in them and they can't. I just say to them, "Try your best because you have got it in you and you can do it. You'll benefit out of it once you leave school. If you don't try and the end of it you end up as a shop assistant", I say, "you've got no-one but yourself to blame".'

The moral significance of work lies chiefly in the fact that it is thought that individuals have the choice, not about whether or not they will be successful – but about whether or not they make the most of themselves and act 'responsibly'. In order to be respectable and respected, people are expected to work hard and to be seen to be working hard to make the most of themselves and their natural advantages, or to put it another way, to overcome their natural disadvantages. For men, this requires having a job and is directly related to the question of employment. For women, it is a different matter altogether. Women's 'real' work is defined as housework and childcare and is never not there to be done. The requirement of women, therefore, is that they should be seen to run their domestic affairs competently.

The other side of the moral evaluation of work is that not working, either because one has no work to do or is not seen to be doing the work one ought to be doing, becomes suspect. Conditions of all kinds that place people outside work have the potential for discrediting them. If a person is retired, or if they are prevented from working by accident or illness, they are less vulnerable to moral condemnation than if they are unemployed or have physical difficulties that are not apparent. Nevertheless, even when a person is retired or obviously ill, it is important for them, and for others talking about them, to establish their credentials as (previously) good workers and as people who have never not been willing to work. The need to show that one is at all times ready and willing to work affects the way in which the people involved in the study react to signs of illness in themselves and others, as well as the way in which they think and talk about illness, and is discussed in Chapter 5.

Unemployment is the worst experience, in the sense of being the most morally reprehensible of all the conditions that place people outside work. It poses a threat to their integrity because it is not automatically assumed that they are unemployed through no fault of their own. On the contrary, the automatic assumption is that it probably is their fault that they are not working and they prefer being on the dole (scrounging). The mass unemployment of recent years has begun to blur the previously clear-cut distinction between the employed and the unemployed, which was based on recognition of two different moral types. But none of the men in the study wanted to be associated with unemployment, and none of the women wanted men in their families to be associated with it either. The questions asked about whether a person was or ever had been unemployed were generally greeted with hostility and resentment, as if the question itself was insulting. Often people answered with statements, disassociating themselves and their relatives from any mention of unemployment at all:

Mick Chalmers: 'I've never drew dole money since I left school.'
Daniel Mayes: 'I've never been to the labour exchange in my life.'

Ben Knight: 'Personally, I don't worry about anything and work don't worry me because I know that if I got the sack tomorrow, I know that I should go to work somewhere else right away.'

Illness can threaten a person's reputation if it stops him or her from working, but the threat it poses is different and less direct than the threat of unemployment. If the illness is not apparent and there are no tangible signs that it renders the person incapable of work, it is likely that he or she will be cast as a malingerer and a hypochondriac and blamed for not working. If the illness is apparent and there are tangible signs of it, then the person is unlikely to be blamed for not working. They will, however, be blamed if it is thought that they are personally implicated in the cause of the illness, i.e. if the illness is their fault. As far as the judgments about other people's integrity are concerned, there are two aspects of illness that count: one is the extent to which it is obviously incapacitating, the other is the commonsense theory about what has caused the illness to occur. For the moment it is sufficient to point out that illness can be a factor in the moral judging that goes on between people if it affects a person's reputation in relation to work. Chapter 5 examines the implications of the relationship between work, reputations, and illness for the ways in which people think about and discuss health and illness. Chapter 6 explores the significance of these themes for their theories about the causes of illness.

Public and private accounts of work

The accounts people gave of their working experience in the interviews should be placed in the context of the preceding discussion about the moral significance of work. Just as there are public and private accounts of community and of what it is like to live in Bethnal Green, so there are public and private accounts of work and of what it is to have a job. Both types of account have in common the fact that it is taken for granted that men and women have to work. There is no question in either of them of people allowing the possibility that they might not work or of them thinking that work, in the abstract rather than particular kinds of work, is not something that ought to be valued.

The public accounts of work reproduce the (ideological) sets of meanings associated with particular types of work which are common social currency; they are not personal accounts of what it is like to do a particular kind of work or to have a certain job. For example, definitions of levels of skill are associated with particular sets of meanings. In the popular imagination, 'skilled' work is associated with images that have been created in and have emerged out of workers' struggles to have their jobs defined as 'skilled' – images of creativity and craftsmanship, of apprenticeship and application, of masters and boys, which are bound up with other images of maleness and brotherhood and respectability. The images provide the meanings that individuals draw upon in public accounts of work to legitimate what they do, as well as to make sense of it to themselves and to other people. Their public accounts of work do not represent the totality of their feelings about work and they do not convey what it is like to do the work, but by validating some aspects of the job and discounting others they outline a relationship to work that others recognise and will accept as legitimate.

The private accounts of work in the interviews usually emerged out of detailed and specific discussion about particular jobs. In them people spoke from their experience about the meaning work holds for them, personally. The distinction between the two types of account is clearer in principle than it is in practice. Essentially it is a post-facto distinction which allows us to identify and explain contradictions in the way people talk about work. We know from other studies (Goldthorpe *et al.* 1968) that it is unusual for people to voice general criticisms or to say that they dislike their work in public without feeling that it will reflect badly on them. But this is a reference to public accounts of work and to the ways in which people identify with their work and legitimate what they do. At other times and in other contexts the same people will talk about their work completely differently, giving private accounts that will include descriptions of the alienation they experience at work and of their attempts to free themselves from its constraints.

The men's public accounts of work in this study were organized around an opposition between external as opposed to intrinsic rewards. The external rewards are chiefly money and security of income, although status and terms of contract including holidays can be included also. Intrinsic rewards are the content of the work and the personal satisfaction derived from doing it. Imagining a hypothetical continuum with external rewards at one end and intrinsic rewards at the other, the public accounts of work of unskilled and semi-skilled workers tended to fall at the external rewards end whilst the public accounts of skilled and professional workers fell at the other.

Mick Chalmers has done manual work since he left school. He is part-trained in a variety of jobs but has mostly been employed to do unskilled and semi-skilled work. He has never not worked and has had 'hundreds of jobs', but he also feels that he has never had a choice about the nature of the work that he does. The only qualification he needs for his present job as a drayman is physical fitness and strength. Mick maintains that the external rewards of work are all that matters:

> JC: 'What does work mean to you?'
> MC: 'The end product, the money.'
> JC: 'That's all? But you said you get bored if you don't go to work.'
> MC: 'Oh yes, it's something to do as well. But I don't actually go to do something. I mean, if they said to me, "There's going to be no money at the end of the week", I definitely wouldn't go and do this job.'

As far as his public account of work is concerned, there is very little Mick can say other than that he does it for the money. In the past he has been uniquely concerned with the amount he was earning and he was willing to do jobs that were dangerous and unpleasant provided they paid well enough. He spent a year digging the Blackwall Tunnel, for example, and in that time two men on his shift were killed. Recently, security of income has become more of a priority for him; he moved to his present job with the brewery because he believed (wrongly as it turns out) that the brewery's future was guaranteed, and that he would have a secure job, if not until he was retired, at least until his children were old enough to go to work. Mick is basically ambivalent about being a labourer. At one time he had been urged by his doctor to give up being a drayman and find work that was less strenuous; the doctor suggested working for the Post Office. But Mick had felt that working for the Post Office was not 'proper work' and that he liked 'doing something where I'm working', meaning doing manual work. On the other hand, in his interview he remarked that he would: 'love to be able to go and do an office job. I'd love to put on a suit and tie and walk into work and sit in an office.'

Daniel Mayes's public account of his work is the account of a skilled man and is very different from Mick's. Daniel maintains that as a skilled wood-machinist he found his job satisfying and pleasurable, and that a man should judge his work not by its external rewards but by the satisfaction it affords him:

'No, money's never been important to me. Not, I think I liked what I was doing, I enjoyed it. If I didn't like it, I wouldn't do it. If you can enjoy what you're doing it's all right. You can go out and earn £30 a week more and every Monday when you get up you think, "Christ, I'm going back there again". You walk in on a Monday morning and you're expecting trouble and what's going to go wrong now? All you've got to look forward to is an extra £30 a week and £20 of that you're going to spend on booze to forget that you've been at work that week. It's just frustration and you don't want frustration when you're working.'

Discounting the financial rewards in itself makes Daniel's job appear in a better light, but he is able to say that money is no object partly because he has not had financial worries for many years, and partly because there are aspects of his job about which he can be positive. In the time that he was employed he was promoted from the shop floor to the level of supervisor; there was some variety in the work; he was able to see projects through from the start to finish and he was in charge of other men.

If what people say about work in public accounts is to be seen as part of a process of legitimation and not simply an expression of their individual attitudes and preferences, it follows that the public accounts of people who have moved from one *type* of work to another are of particular interest. The changes registered in their accounts might of course be nothing more than the attitudinal changes that can occur in the course of one individual's lifetime, but there are indications that they are basically occasioned by the individuals in question having an adaptable response to novel situations and adopting the public account that goes with the job. Ben Knight, for example, first worked for London Transport because, to his knowledge, it had a reputation for paying well. He had no special inclination to be a bus driver, but according to his account, *at that time* he had a wife and child to support and money was his first priority. It might well be argued that money remained his priority and that he sensibly chose to work in Billinsgate where the chances of making money through his own initiative were far greater than his chances of making money in London Transport ever could have been. However, he recalls his swich from one job to another as a change in priorities, away from external rewards and towards a life at work that was intrinsically more interesting. He now insists that he is not 'a well-paid man', and that money matters less than job satisfaction:

> 'No-one can really buy you off, money is not the name of the game virtually. It is in the end product, but it's satisfaction at work, you know. A lot of people will take a little less money and be more satisfied at a job than someone who's got to work terrible hard and never be satisfied.'

William Cox has moved in the opposite direction to Ben Knight, away from the intrinsic rewards of skilled work and towards the greater financial rewards of (in this case) manual labour. William turned to labouring when he was unable to find enough work as an electrician to support his family. Having made that shift he is less concerned to support the idea that skilled work is necessarily more rewarding than other work than he is to emphasize the importance of money.

The two men in the group who do semi-skilled work and are badly paid – Stan Flowers and Joe Hutchinson – gave brief public accounts of their work without much conviction. Both men simply said that they work to get paid, with Stan adding that he liked to work because it gave him something to do. Their talk about work resembled the women's talk in this respect. Most of the women are semi-skilled or unskilled and badly paid and, like the two men, there was nothing positive they could say in public about their jobs. However, not having a public account mattered less to them because their identity was less at stake in talking about work. They explicitly related their paid work to economic necessity and to the needs of the household in general, rather than to themselves. Most of them were reticent about housework and childcare, however, which does constitute their 'real' work. In the same way that Stan and Joe seemed to feel that there was nothing much they could say about their work, the women had nothing to say about housework other than that 'it had to be done'.

The differences between the men and the women in relation to work were apparent in their private accounts of their experience of work. All of them, men and women alike, were preoccupied with the twin issues of authority and control in the workplace, but in different ways and for different reasons. It seemed important for the men to be able to say that they 'were somebody' at work, that they were 'free' and that they were able also to 'be their own boss'.

Their relationship to work is fundamentally contradictory in the sense that they both believe it to be true that people get what they deserve (they are what they are meant to be) and know from their experience that the alternatives available to them personally have been limited. They resolve the contradiction subjectively by dwelling on aspects of their work that they can represent as allowing them to be autonomous in their workplace. Ben Knight and Daniel Mayes both drew attention to the intrinsic rewards of their jobs in their public accounts, but made it clear in private accounts that the source of their satisfaction lay not in the content of the work itself but in the fact that there was no-one above them telling them what to do. Daniel Mayes had hoped that the work itself would have a creative element, but it was basically routine and undemanding. He enjoyed using his skills at home to make furniture and toys, but at work his chief satisfaction came from being able to come and go as he pleased and from having the feeling that his employers respected him:

'But the nice part about it was I didn't have the governor come and tell me what to do. He would come and say to me, "Daniel, do you think you could do this?" which was nice. I won't be told that, "You will get that out", you see. It was my mill, I was in charge of the mill and that was it.'

Stan Flowers and Mick Chalmers are manual labourers with no authority at work. Questions of how they are treated at work and of who controls their time are, if anything, more important to them precisely because they are not in charge of what they are doing. The reason Stan had stayed with his most recent employers was that they had consulted him when they wanted to put him on short-time, and had given him the feeling that they had some respect for him as a person. Mick Chalmers stayed in his job with the brewery because, in comparison with other jobs he had had, it allowed him to feel that he was in charge of himself whilst he was working:

'At the moment, I like the job, I do like the job. I get out, I get about. I'm not stuck in one place all the time and I'm me own boss. I ain't got nobody over me. I ain't being told what to do and what not to do. Once I go in, we load the lorry up and go out on the road, it's just the three of us. We can stop when we like, have a drink when we like, have something to eat. It's not really a bad job when you look at it that way. I'm not being hassled by a foreman and having to answer to anybody. Once I'm on the road, I'm me own governor.'

Both men spoke of their time as precious, and yet when they were not at work (and both spent substantial periods of time at home, Stan because he worked three days a week, Mick because he usually left work at midday after an early start), they find that time hangs heavily on their hands, that they are bored and restless and sometimes feel depressed, and are at a loss to know what to do with themselves. The significance of time and of having control over their own time in relation to work was that both of them had a sense of having won something from a situation in which they normally expect to lose.

In contrast with the men's need to feel respected and to be in charge at work, at least of themselves, the women's interest in the issues of authority and control in the workplace stemmed from a desire to have a 'good time' and to be free to relate to other people at work. They experienced their domestic obligations as the source of subjection to authority, control, and lack of freedom in their lives, and having a job was in itself a welcome release from them. Their comparisons between different jobs were based on the quality of the 'atmosphere' and whether or not they liked the people they worked with:

'It's no good working in a place where the atmosphere is wrong. They weren't good payers. It was in Hackney Road, I could've gone on up Liverpool Street two stops and possibly got £30 more, but as I said to him [William Cox], he said, "You're mad. What are you working round here for, for that?" I said, "Yes, I know, Will. But the thing is, it's no good going two stops up the road, £30 more, when you hate the place."'

The women varied according to which aspects of their jobs they emphasized as the more important. Ann Cullen, for example, was preoccupied with the content of the actual work and the discomfort of doing it, but she works more than the other women and always has done:

'When you say to people, "I'm a machinist", "Oh, that's a cushy job. You're sitting down all day." But it's not as simple as that. You get backache, your legs ache. If you're a piece-worker you've got to earn your money and you've got a bit of hard work. It takes from the time you go in, you're on the go until you're finished.'

At the other extreme, Ann's sister, Betty, and Mary Webb, both of whom did a few hours' office cleaning, were principally concerned with whether or not they had a good time whilst they were at work:

> Betty: 'I think that's what you go to work for, to be amongst people. You have a laugh, have a joke. You see a lot of women that don't go to work, they let theirselves go. They think to themselves "I ain't got to wash meself up because I'm going nowhere". When you go to work you know you've got to get up, wash yourself and dress yourself.'
> JC: 'Is that why you go to work now?'
> BM: 'Yes, I like going to work.'
> JC: 'Do you feel different at work from at home?'
> BM: 'Yes, I think you feel different in yourself.'
> JC: 'What's the differrence?'
> BM: 'I don't know, you go to work to have a laugh. You come home, do your work and that's it.'

Sarah Chalmers falls somewhere between the two extremes. She does part-time work in local factories, working as a machinist, a packer and an assembly worker. Since she went back to work after having her children she has never not had a job, but she changes from one job to another regularly whenever she gets bored or dislikes someone or stops enjoying herself.

Thus there were differences in the way the men and the women involved in the study talked about their work, in their feelings about work and in the meanings that work had for them. Townsend's research into the condition of old people in Bethnal Green (1957) and the interview material concerning old people in the study families suggests that the differences persist into retirement. Men generally seem to find retirement much harder to cope with than women. Townsend described the men he met as engaged 'in a rather desperate search for pastimes or a gloomy contemplation of their own helplessness which, at its worst, was little better than waiting to die' (1957: 169). Women, on the other hand, having always identified more with domestic life than with paid work, do not have the experience of breaking with the main activity which has not only taken up most of their time but has also been their chief source of identity, that men have and they tend to look forward more to retirement and to enjoy it. In comparison with the men, they seem more able to use their time in a way that is satisfying. They never stop working completely.

'Even Nellie Davies, who did very little housework, was more active in the house – making tea and sandwiches, washing-up, and writing out lists of shopping for other people to do – than her husband, who did nothing except watch the television and wait for opening time at the pub. Yet more important is the fact that the women tend to see more of other people than the men. There are, of course, old women who are incapacitated and house-bound, and women who have been single all their lives or who have no relatives who are close to them, who find old age and retirement as difficult and as lonely as the older men in the study families. But in general, the early lives of the women seem to equip them to survive old age less unhappily than the men, principally because they are more sociable and remain involved with other people.

Conclusion

In conclusion to this discussion of work and attitudes towards work it may be useful to re-emphasize some of the points relevant to the discussions of health and illness and health services in later chapters. The principal attitude towards work amongst people involved in the study that this chapter has described is one which attaches great importance to the part the individual must play in determining his or her own lot in life. This at least was the message in the public accounts of work that were examined, although the private accounts of work told a somewhat different story. The reality the private accounts described was one of little choice and of no room to take individual action in the way that public accounts suggest is a possibility. In private accounts it was clearly much more a question of adapting positively to circums-tances – of 'making the best of it' rather than 'making the most of oneself'. There is a direct parallel between the different positions the two types of account describe in relation to work and the different positions in public and private accounts of health and illness that we will come to later (see Chapters 5 and 6).

It is relevant to note also with respect to the differences between the two types of account of work, the close correspondence between the attitudes and values expressed in public accounts, and the attitudes and values of the popular press and of ministers in the present government towards 'scrounging', unemployment, the importance of showing individual initiative, and so on. It is not possible in a study such as this accurately to trace the origins of particular ideologies, but it seems likely that the individualism one might associate with East London industrial traditions – with the 'calling on' system of casual labour on the docks and the large industrial sector made up of small manufacturing enterprises – has been twisted into new shape by the economic philosophy of the current conservative majority. Once again, it can be seen that experts of various kinds – in this case politicians, political commentators, monetarist economists, and the press – influence the content of the commonsense ideas and theories that dominate public accounts. The importance of 'experts' and of expert opinion is a theme that is taken up in relation to doctors and the medical profession in the chapters that are concerned with health and illness and the health services.

Finally, it remains to draw attention to the differences between the sexes which have been noted in this chapter and to their relevance for the discussions about health matters generally in chapters to follow. We have seen that men and women in the study have different attitudes towards employment and very different working experience, and that the relationship of women to employment is determined by their primary responsibility for housework and childcare. The next chapter examines more closely the domestic division of labour and the ideology that legitimates it.

4 Family Life

Introduction

Almost everything about the way the men and women in this study lead their lives is different. Some differences have been alluded to in earlier chapters. We know, for example, that the men and women who were approached to take part in the study responded differently, with the men in general being more reluctant, and we know also that the content of their interviews was different. The interviews showed that men and women had a different perspective on 'community', different relationships with their neighbours, and also a different relationship to paid work. So far, the subject of sexual difference has been raised but has not been closely examined, and yet it is of great significance for the relationship that people in the study have with their health and with the health services. There are, for example, differences in the way men and women respond to symptoms and cope with feeling unwell, differences in the extent of their responsibilities for their own and other people's health, and differences in their use of health services and in their information about health and illness and about the health services.

The aim in this chapter is to examine the differences in more detail and to try to explain the basis for them. The theoretical perspective adopted is one that attributes the differences between men and women to their respective structural positions in relation to production and reproduction, i.e., to differences in their access to and control over resources in these two areas. We have seen in Chapter 3 that the local labour market in East London is sexually segregated and is particularly disadvantageous for women. Local men and women are in a different position with regard to employment, with women's jobs concentrated in unskilled, low-paid positions in industries where the working conditions are poor and there is very little or no job security. It has been intimated that both the men and the women involved in the study took it for granted that their position in relation to paid work should be different, because to them the 'real' work that women do – and that they expect women to put before their paid jobs – is their work at home. The domestic division of labour in most of the study families is entirely traditional, with the women having responsibility for the housework and childcare and the men occasionally helping out and playing with the children. The division of labour is legitimated on biological grounds, the argument being that the differences between men and women are natural in the sense that they stem from their respective reproductive roles. Ultimately, therefore, the belief in women's domesticity, which legitimates the sexual division of labour in the study families, is based on beliefs about the primacy of reproductive roles and functions.

The question we need to ask, of course, is why is it like that? Why are the social and economic lives of the men and women in the study families principally defined by their biological functions? Why is the sexual division of labour in these families so rigid and traditional? Some answers are supplied by other studies where there seems to be general agreement that the character of the social and economic environment in East London is particularly conducive to a traditional sexual division of labour and thus to sexual segregation between men and women in the same families. The relative geographical immobility of the people involved in the study (many of their relatives have been dispersed but those that remain in East London move very little), the lack of occupational diversity amongst the men coupled with a superior earning capacity which gives them virtually absolute economic control over their immediate family, and the relative lack of (good) job opportunities for women are all contributory factors (Harris 1969; Bott 1957; Morpeth and Langton 1974; Frankenberg 1976).

The analysis in this chapter suggests relationships between these and other factors, such as the availability of housing for single parents and the availability of information about and access to methods of birth control, all of which are extraordinarily complex and difficult to unravel. The number of children per family in Bethnal Green has diminished sharply over the last few decades (Gittins 1982), but most people in the study married and had children in their early twenties (if not before), and before they had time to secure any measure of financial or social independence from their families of origin. It was not unusual, as we know already, for couples to start married life in their parents' home. The economic, occupational, and psychological consequences of youthful parenthood for women are more dramatic than for men because of the meanings that are attached to motherhood. Women with children are expected to make their children's needs their first priority, which basically means that they are expected to be at home looking after the children full-time, especially during the period when the children are too young to go to school. Automatically, then, the women lose their immediate opportunities for further education and training, and the long-term effects on their employment prospects are such that they are, as they see themselves to be, dependent on their men. It is not possible to find out from the research interviews why the men and women in these families marry and have children (or, often, have children and marry) when they are still only in their teens and early twenties. Amongst the adults in the youngest generation involved in the study, all the first pregnancies were accidental. This does not necessarily mean that they were unwanted, but they led straight into early marriage. It is for that reason that contraception and housing allocations policy are both factors in the over-all picture of the unequal sexual division of labour which is the focus for discussion in this chapter.

The approach to family life in this chapter is similar to that adopted in the previous two chapters. A case study of one extended family network – the Davies family – provides the empirical back-drop to a discussion of the two different types of account of family life contained in the interviews. The motivation underlying the public accounts was clearly that of wanting to say the 'right' and acceptable thing, but it was apparent also that their content expressed needs which people had that were not fulfilled in the way in which they actually led their lives. The images of family life in public accounts were images of unity, of men and women and different generations of relatives having loving relationships that were personally satisfying and essentially 'good'. The private accounts told a different story. They drew attention, often humourously, to the strain family life imposes on the individual members of families and to the contradictions that led to an absence of relating and to relationships that were full of overt and unexpressed conflict.

The concluding section of the chapter is devoted to a further, fairly lengthy contribution to the critique of Young and Willmott (1957) started in Chapter 2. The fact that the two studies have been conducted in the same area and that there is a period of almost thirty years between them makes a comparison between them intrinsically worth doing. It is interesting to look back to Young and Willmott's study to see how accurate they have been in the predictions they made about the future of the family in Bethnal Green, and about the direction of some of the changes that they believed were taking place at the time when they were writing. More importantly, their interpretation of family life in Bethnal Green has become very widely known amongst both academic and lay audiences and has been accepted – in much the same way as their portrait of Bethnal Green was accepted as the model modern urban village – as an account of family life not just in Bethnal Green but in the working class generally. The particular significance of this is that their interpretation can be faulted on both theoretical and methodological grounds and yet it has been taken up and used quite uncritically by sociologists working in other fields, including medical sociology. Thus many of the assumptions in the medical sociological literature about why working class people use health services differently from middle class people are derived from Young and Willmott's interpretation of the character and quality of relationships in working class families (see, for instance, McKinlay 1970; 1973). For this reason it has been considered especially important to look back at their work and to draw attention to the analytical and interpretive differences between *Family and Kinship* and the present study.

The Davies family: a case study

Nellie Davies was eighty when she was interviewed; a year older than her husband, Arthur, who was in hospital at the time. She and Arthur first met during the First World War in a khaki clothing factory. Arthur had been fourteen when the war started, too young to become a soldier, but old enough to do war work. They married after the war ended, when Nellie was twenty, Arthur nineteen.

They spent the first years of their married lives in Nellie's parent's house, where they had one room for themselves and their growing number of children. Nellie had eleven children in all – seven girls and four boys – six of whom were born whilst they were still living with her parents. At the time of the interviews, nine of Nellie's children were alive, all seven of her daughters and her two younger sons. Nellie's eldest son died three years before the study began of cancer of the liver; he was fifty-five. Her third son is also dead. He died of pneumonia in infancy.

In 1930, Nellie and Arthur moved from her parents' house into one of their own in Bethnal Green, where she subsequently had the five younger children. Between 1939 and 1945, the whole family was separated and dispersed around the country. Arthur and his older boy were called up; Nellie, the two eldest girls, the two remaining sons, and the youngest daughter who was only three when the war began stayed in Bethnal Green, and the four middle daughters were evacuated to different parts of the country. After the war, the family re-assembled in a different house (their old home had suffered severe bomb damage), a large Victorian terraced house on four floors.

As the daughters grew up, all of them with the exception of Kathleen (see page 34) lived with their husbands and first children in the house, until they either managed to find somewhere of their own to rent or were allocated a house or flat by the local council. Joan Young lived with her parents the longest; it was nine years before she eventually moved to a flat of her own, by which time she had two children. Nellie and Arthur's sons did not live at home after they were married. One moved straight into his parents-in-law's house after getting married, the others moved with their wives into rented accommodation. For a short time after the children had all grown up they lived within two square miles of Nellie and Arthur, but in the mid nineteen-fifties three of the daughters moved with their families to New Towns in the South East and Kathleen moved to Dagenham where she spent two years before coming back to Bethnal Green. Since then the youngest of the seven daughters has moved out of Bethnal Green, and now lives with her family in Essex.

When Nellie's daughters were younger and still living locally, they all visited her every day with or without their children. In doing so, they stayed in close contact with each other even after they had left home. Often Nellie cooked a midday meal for all of them as well as for Arthur and her sons, who ate at home at midday rather than going home to their wives. Nellie provided innumerable services for her daughters as they established themselves in their own households with their husbands and children. The daughters left their children with her when they wanted to shop, or if they had an appointment to attend, and when they went to work; they relied on Nellie to pass word to their sisters if they were ill or needed help from them, either with the housework or with looking after the children; they asked Nellie's advice about what to do when the children were ill and about whether or not to consult a doctor for them; often they took husbands and children to Nellie's house at weekends and she provided meals for all of them.

As the daughters' children – Nellie's grandchildren – grew older and started going to school, the daughters became able to arrange employment for themselves around the children's hours at school. Some of the daughters had left the area altogether, and they and Nellie began to see less of each other. The daughters still relied on her, and increasingly on each other, for help if they were ill and in other emergencies, but instead of all visiting Nellie every day, they made arrangements with each other to visit separately so that, between them, they would cover the week. Gradually the balance began to shift, and it was them helping Nellie rather than Nellie helping them. Each daughter started doing some service or other for Nellie when they paid her a visit. One did the shopping; another vacuumed the carpets; another changed the bed-linen; another took the washing to the launderette; and so on. Eventually, between them, they had taken over all the household chores and there was nothing left for Nellie to do, other than prepare meals and write out shopping lists for other people. But having started out with good intentions of wanting their mother to be able to take life a little more easily and wanting to repay her for her hard work on their behalf, the daughters began to regret their actions. In their interviews, Joan, Kathleen, and Mary said that the arrangement had turned out badly for all of them. It had created a vacuum in Nellie's life, and not knowing what else she could do with herself, she had become increasingly preoccupied with her own physical ailments and was now a fully-fledged hypochondriac. Meanwhile, they are finding that as they grow older, their responsibilities and involvements with their own children and grandchildren use up most of their energy, and their obligations towards their mother are increasingly burdensome:

KR: 'With Mum, she's sort of enjoyed bad health. I know it sounds wicked, but still she has, over the last few years. And even if, I've noticed that she talks to her sisters on the phone, I'm going back a few months now, she's as right as rain. If she was to talk to Millie [the eldest daughter] on the phone, "Oh, I do feel ill. I'm this, I'm that", and that's in the same afternoon. It

depends on who she's talking to for feeling ill or feeling well . . .
Not so much look after her, but she wants you to feel sorry for
her. All right, at the back of our minds we probably all do feel
sorry for her because she's had such a hard life really. But she
don't make matters any easier by trying to cope for herself. All
right, as me brother said, we've made it worse because we've
done too much for her, and we've made life boring for her so
that all she had to do was sit and think about her health.'

Nellie and Arthur stopped talking to each other (beyond the
minimal exchanges that automatically take place between two
people who share the same roof) almost three years before the
study started, but none of their children remembers them ever
having had much to do with each other. Nellie was always at
home with the children and Arthur was always out – working or
just out. The daughters do not remember their parents either
going out on their own together or going out with the children.
The most Joan could say about her parents' relationship was that
her father has never been violent towards Nellie, although
Kathleen recalled angry scenes between the two of them over
Arthur's earnings and the amount he allowed Nellie for house-
keeping. The following passage from an interview with Kathleen
conveys much of the quality of their relationship in recent years:

'I think you might as well turn round and say that I think it's
since he retired they've not really communicated. They went
through a little spell of it. That's when she sort of done her nut
about "he's out at the pub every night" and this, that and the
other. But it's because he got fed up of asking her to go out of a
night. I said, "Don't moan about it because he's offered to take
you, so if you prefer to sit indoors on your own, that's up to
you". Well, she must have thought, because we all more or less
said the same thing, 'cause everyone who was going in was
saying she was moaning about him going down to the pub and
she was stuck in of a night waiting for him to come in. And we'd
all more or less said the same. "You had your chance, you
should have gone with him." Well, he still didn't give up. He
still used to ask, and then one day he got so annoyed he
shoved her coat on and said, "Get your coat on, get out".
Anyway, she was going out for quite a long while after that but,
as I say, it's over two years she stopped going out. She just
reckoned she didn't feel well, she didn't feel well enough, he
stopped asking. Still, you can't blame him. I think that he's not

so much deaf now, it's just that he's shut himself off from her, and he's shut himself off from us, unless you shout first to let him know you're talking to him, and then he'll hold a conversation quite easily, if he knows you're talking to him. But apart from that, he'll just sit in his chair, shut his earholes off of everything.'

Compared with the women, the men play a very small part in the immediate and the extended family. Nellie and Arthur's sons seem to have played different roles in the family. The elder one, now dead, was his parents' favourite and popular with all his sisters. From his sisters' reports of him, he never took much part in the practical affairs of the others – he left that to his sisters – but they all saw him regularly and often, and he was the one who organized family get-togethers and parties. The younger brothers have always had very little to do with the family. They visit their parents occasionally but do not arrange their visits with their sisters, as they arrange theirs with each other. Their sisters talk of them much as they talk of strangers.

The daughters' husbands have, with one exception, had little to do with Nellie and Arthur or with other members of the family, despite having spent in some cases years under the same roof as them. The exception is Joan's husband, Patrick, who for a while became closely involved in nursing and generally helping out after Arthur had one leg amputated. The fact that it was Patrick rather than any of the other sons-in-law was purely a matter of convenience. He lived the closest and, because he was on short-time working, had the time to take on these extra responsibilities. Once Arthur was able to manage again on his own, the two saw as little of each other as they had done previously.

The daughters' husbands rarely spend much time with members of their immediate families, and the part they play in domestic life at home is relatively small. Kathleen's first husband was a coach driver. He left home early in the morning, and at weekends and on summer evenings was usually out fishing. He had been very close to his mother, whom Kathleen disliked, and he spent more time with her than he did with Kathleen and his children. Kathleen's second husband, Stan, and Joan's husband, Patrick, are both wood-workers with similar life-styles. When they are not working, both of them spend their evenings and much of the weekend at the local pub or at the working men's club. On average, they are at home for one evening a week, which they spend in front of the television. When Stan was interviewed, he was on short-time work and was at home for at least two days of the working week. He said that he hated being at home and had no idea what to do with himself. Mary's husband, Charlie Webb, is self-employed and works very long hours and regularly a seven-day week.

Nellie's daughters all have children and five of them, including Kathleen and Mary, are grandmothers as well as having children still at home. Their relationships with their daughters who have children are not unlike the relationships they themselves had with Nellie when they were young mothers. They provide the back-up service that Nellie provided for them. Kathleen's eldest daughter, Sharon, lived with Kathleen for the first few months after she was married and then moved into a flat of her own. During the first few months after her first child was born she spent all day, every day with Kathleen whom she relied on totally for help with the baby:

> 'I used to depend on Mum a lot. And after I had him, I didn't have a clue. And having her so close as well, downstairs, she used to do all the washing as well. I used to take all me washing to her . . . She did, she used to do all the washing and all the ironing as well. I don't think I did a thing. All I was doing was cooking when I got home.'

Sharon eventually mastered looking after the baby on her own, but she continued to visit Kathleen every day and to spend the day with her until she decided to go back to work and leave him with his grandmother altogether. Now that she is at work, she relies on Kathleen to take him to school in the morning and to look after him if he is unwell and cannot attend school.

Kathleen's second daughter, Joanne, has been even more dependent than Sharon on her mother for help with her children. When her two eldest children were still very young, the local social services wanted to take them away from her and have them put into care, at which point Kathleen offered to foster them. The children stayed with Kathleen for nearly two years, during which time Joanne visited most days and at the week end. They then returned home to live with their mother, but Kathleen continues to feel responsible for their welfare and she takes an active part in looking after them and their younger brother. She takes and fetches them from school and the children stay and play at her house after school until Joanne comes and fetches them. Often they have their evening meal at Kathleen's house and she cooks Sunday dinners for them as well. She also frequently baby-sits for Joanne who is now a single parent.

Mary Webb's daughter, Nicola, gave birth to Mary's first grandchild in the course of the study. In the first weeks of the baby's life, Nicola called on Mary many times throughout the day for reassurance about the baby and for help with washing, shopping, ironing, and cooking. Mary's third interview took place four weeks after Nicola had the baby and was interrupted by a phone call from Nicola's husband that was typical of the inter-action between the two households in that period. The phone call was to ask Mary to pop in later in the morning because Nicola was worried about the baby who had a heat rash.

'He said, "I should have phoned earlier", he said, "but I did and there was no answer". He must have phoned when I was taking Ben to school . . . She doesn't know whether to take him to the doctor's or to the clinic, or what. But more than likely he's – he's immuned at the moment anyway from measles and things like that so I think it's just a heat rash even without going up there . . . But normally he phones me up. He phoned me up on Monday. "Can you go up and see Nicola, she's had no sleep all night long" he's going. "I'm ever so worried about her." This is David. I said, "Yes, I'll pop up." And so I did. As soon as I took Ben to school I popped up there and she did look exhausted.'

Mary and Kathleen have very little to do with their sons-in-law, although both of them have had them living under the same roof with them. Kathleen rarely sees Sharon's husband and hardly knows him. If she sees him at all, it is because Sharon has sent him around to help her with an odd job of some kind, such as helping to fit a new ceiling light, or checking leaking pipes. Mary sees equally little of her son-in-law, and makes a point of not being there with Nicola once he is at home. The daughters visit their mothers rather than the mothers visiting the daughters, precisely to avoid involving them with their husbands.

Both Sharon and Nicola, and Joanne who is now divorced, met their husbands when they were at school, and all of them were pregnant before they were married. Sharon and Nicola's husbands spend more time at home than the older men in the family. They work shorter hours, although Nicola's husband is a car worker and works shifts, and they go out less often because they are trying to save money to buy their own homes. When they are at home, they occasionally take the children out or play with them indoors, but neither of them shares the housework. Most of their time at home is spent sleeping or watching television.

There are many ways in which the Davies family as a whole, and the different generations within it, resemble other families, involved in the study. Before the war, Bethnal Green had one of the highest birth-rates in England and Wales (although it was also declining more sharply than the birth-rate anywhere else in the country (Gittins 1982)) and it was not unusual either for pre-war families in Bethnal Green to be very large, or for some of the children to die when they were young. Ann Cullen and Betty Mayes came from a family of seventeen children, two of whom died in infancy. Harold and Florrie Neagle had twelve children, of whom only nine survived. Ben Knight came from a family of six children.

Where different generations of the same family live close together, the relations between mothers and daughters are similar to the relationships between Nellie and her daughters, Kathleen and Mary, and between Kathleen and Mary and *their* daughters. When their mother was alive, Ann Cullen and Betty Mayes used to see all their brothers and sisters every week, some of them every day, but since first she and then their father died, they have seen less of their siblings. Ann sees this as proof that mothers hold families together:

'When me mother was alive, every Saturday they was up to see her, so of course you see them. But then when me Mum died, for a while they still come up to see me Dad, but then it gradually drifted off, which I think happens in most families. Because then when me Mum died, I think it just automatically goes that way, and I think this happens in most families. Once the parents are gone, you don't seem to see so much of each other.'

Ann now sees her daughter, Jackie, every day, twice a day, once in the morning on her way to work and again in the evening on her way home. She and Jackie also visit Betty on two or three afternoons a week on their way home from picking up Jackie's daughters from school. All three women do their shopping together on Saturdays. Sarah Chalmers is older than Jackie, and her children are all in secondary school. Her mother lives across the road from her and she has one sister who lives nearby. She sees her mother almost every day and does odd bits of shopping for her, and often sees her sister when she calls in at her mother's. Sarah's husband, Mick, sees his mother-in-law very rarely, even though he lives across the street from her.

There are also clear similarities between the relationships between men and women in the Davies family and in other families. Harold and Florrie Neagle argue and row with one another constantly, and Harold spends every evening out, either at the pub or at his friends, the McInneses, to avoid his wife's company. With the exception of two men, the men of the middle generation spend very little time with their wives and children, and even less with the members of their own and their wives' extended families. The exceptions are Daniel Mayes and Joe Hutchinson. Daniel likes being at home more than anything else, and unusually for the men, does some of the heavier housework, helping Betty with the shopping and with vacuuming the carpets. Joe Hutchinson is a widower. He has learned to run the house and take care of his children on his own and takes great pleasure in doing so. The other men either work very long hours, as is the case with Eddie Cullen, Ann's husband, or they fill their time with activities that take them away from home, such as fishing, following sport, or drinking.

The men of the younger generation spend variable amounts of time at home. Mick Chalmers is often at home in the afternoons, because he starts work very early. He usually dozes in front of the television and wakes up to go out after his evening meal to the local pub. His wife accompanies him at weekends. William Cox works long hours, often leaving home before six in the morning and coming in late at night. If he does leave work early, he goes to the pub with his father-in-law, Eddie Cullen, with whom he works, and with whom he also drinks at weekends.

Public and private accounts of family life

The public accounts of family life in the interviews tended to be given early on in the interviews and in answer to questions that focussed attention on family relationships. The questions that provoked them were questions such as, "What was your mother/ father like?" "What was your parents' relationship like?" Sometimes people gave a public account of someone in the family or of a particular family relationship if they took the question they had been asked to have implied criticism. For example, most of the women gave public answers to questions about the amount of time their husbands spent at home and the amount that their husbands did of housework or looking after the children, which they contradicted later in their private accounts of the same things.

The public accounts were always concerned with the same, limited aspects of domestic and familial relations, always represented in exactly the same way. The aspects in question were connected to an explicit, specialized division of labour which defined exactly what was expected of men and women in the context of the family. The public accounts also often contained moral judgments which were made on the basis of how well this or that person fulfilled their roles and tasks in the domestic division of labour. Given that one of the chief purposes of public accounts is to legitimate the person who is giving them, public accounts of families – as the people with whom the speaker is likely to be most closely associated – are particularly crucial. Thus, putting the 'best face' on oneself almost invariably became putting the 'best face' on members of one's family. Because public accounts cannot afford to make judgments that might reflect badly on the speaker, most of the judgments people made of the parts they and their relatives played in the family were positive.

In the public accounts of family life in the interviews the family is portrayed as a 'natural' social unit in which the generations and the sexes 'naturally' complement each other. Family life is always represented as something that 'works', with all the qualities of wholeness and integration and of something that is lasting, commonly and popularly associated with the products of nature.

The picture of family life in these accounts is a picture of a traditional domestic division of labour in which men and women are engaged in separate and different activities, in pursuit of the common objective of 'doing the best for the children'. It assumes that the content of what they do in their separate ways is 'naturally', or to be more specific, biologically determined. Women's activities are domestic and include all aspects of maintaining the family and the household: 'caring' for husbands and children in the fullest sense of the word. Men's activities involve the relation between the family and the outside world. They are expected to provide an income that is adequate for the family and for its individual members: at home, they look after the car (if there is one); garden; maintain external appearances – painting and decorating; and are responsible for external amenities – gas, water, electricity.

The belief in female domesticity on which the traditional division of labour rests ultimately reduces to beliefs about motherhood: beliefs that the mother-child relationship is a 'natural unit', and that women have a maternal instinct which makes them more able to take care of children than men could ever be (Oakley 1974: 158). They have their natural corollary in beliefs about men and work: beliefs that men are the 'natural' providers and protectors of the family unit, but that they also need actively to make their mark on the outside world. These assumptions and beliefs have been rejected by feminists who have argued that they justify the exploitation of women as unpaid labourers in the home, and maintain women's unequal position in labour markets (Gardner 1976; Hunt and Hunt 1974), but they are used by both the men and the women involved in the study to make sense of family life.

Their public accounts of family life are not sentimental. They portray marriage as a contract between a man and a woman to do the job of having a family and bringing up children. The definition of whether or not a marriage is successful does not depend on a romantic ideal of husband and wife remaining in love or sustaining a close personal relationship, but on each of them fulfilling their part of the contract. Similarly, the public accounts of other relationships in families and especially of relationships between parents and children are not concerned with levels of personal happiness or intimacy between family members, but with how well people do what is expected of them.

Within the group of people involved in this study there are noticeable differences in the degree to which individuals appear to be personally invested in public accounts of family life, corresponding to differences between the generations. The older people were much less concerned with giving public accounts of their families than were the younger people. The interviews with the older people (i.e. with Nellie Davies and Harold and Florrie Neagle) contained fewer of the stock phrases describing so-and-so as a 'good' mother/father/husband etc. than the other interviews. They contained information about themselves and other relatives that was at odds with the harmonious image of family life promoted in the others' public accounts, and that, in contrast with some of the more guarded responses of the younger people responding to questions about the family, was volunteered freely. The older people also made less of children, and of the importance of doing one's best for them as the principal objective of family life.

There are two alternative explanations for these generational differences. Either the older people are less concerned and feel themselves to be less implicated by public accounts in general, or, in this particular instance, their version of the public account is different. Both are plausible, and with this small number of cases it is not possible to be certain which is the more valid. However, there are grounds for believing that the second is the more likely explanation because generational differences also occur with the public accounts of other subjects, and in some instances there are even generationally different *versions* of public accounts of the same thing (see Chapter 7).

Nellie Davies and the Neagles showed no interest at all in upholding a public account either of their own or of their parents' marriages. Throughout her interview, Nellie Davies grumbled and complained about her husband, insisting that she was not going to run around after him, as he would want her to, when he came out of hospital: 'I'm not doing nothing, he'll have to do it all himself. I can hear him saying, "Do this, do that".' Kathleen Read, Nellie's daughter, who was present at the interview, tried to persuade her mother that 'the poor old soul' (Arthur) was genuinely in pain and had suffered a great deal in having his leg amputated, but Nellie would have none of it. His nerves had always been bad, he kept her awake at night and she never got enough sleep, and she wanted nothing more to do with him: 'I'll bloody divorce him when he comes home. I'll find another old man.' Her threats of divorce were not intended to be taken seriously, but nor was she concerned to create an impression of a marriage that was success-ful, and this embarassed Kathleen. In private accounts, Kathleen and her sisters freely admitted that their parents did not get on with each other, but Kathleen did not want her mother to say so, or at least she did not want this to be all her mother said about it when she was interviewed.

Florrie Neagle described her parents as having always fought 'like cat and dog', both of them regularly drinking to excess. As a child, she had regularly helped her mother undress when she was drunk and put her to bed; she and her mother shared a bed because her father refused to sleep with his wife. Both parents resorted to physical violence to end arguments and Florrie suggested that this had even been the cause of her sister's death:

'My sister, Annie, she died when she was about fourteen months old. But if she would have lived, love, she would have been in a long cane chair, she could never walk. You see, my Mum and Dad used to fight, really fight, because it was, in them days, it was the natural thing for husbands and wives to fight, and they had great families. And my father hit my Mum and caught her in the side. And when my sister was born, she was born with something the matter with her spine. They took her in the London hospital, they couldn't cure her, so she died.'

Having been 'brought up rough', Harold and Florrie did say that they had 'tried to give them [their children] everything they wanted. We did give them everything.' But gambling, physical fights and crime were also important parts of their lives, none of which is compatible with the concern shown elsewhere in public accounts to be acceptable and respectable, and all of which they enjoyed discussing.

Amongst the people in the next generation down from these three it was clearly more important to present a positive view of family life as working. In the context of the interviews this meant emphasizing the efforts that had been made on behalf of children, making explicit positive judgments about all one's relatives (everyone is a 'good' mother/father/husband etc. in their own way), and repudiating the legitimacy of the women working outside the home except as something that is done on behalf of the children. Women's paid employment is an issue in this generation because most of the women are and have been paid workers for substantial periods. Their mothers rarely worked outside the home because they had too many children to look after and jobs were difficult enough for men to find, let alone the women. Their daughters have sometimes worked for a short time before having a first baby and then returned to work part-time, but they are mostly, with the exception of Sarah Chalmers, still at an age where domestic responsibilities take up most of their time. Kathleen Read, Joan Young, Ann Cullen, Betty Mayes and Peggy Freeman have all worked for most of their adult lives, but they represent their work as less important than the 'proper' work they do at home. Mary Webb is the exception in this generation of women in the study. She has eight children and has only started doing part-time work in the last five years since the youngest started school.

The one who had the most difficulty in representing her paid work as 'just a job' was Ann Cullen, because she is the only one who continued to work even when her daughter, Jackie, was a young baby. Ann has spent her entire adult life working and also has a history of very stable employment. She worked for one firm for sixteen years before joining her present firm where she has been for twelve years. Perhaps because of this, of all the women, she was the most concerned to justify her work as having been on Jackie's behalf:

> 'There's only one thing that I always regretted when I had my Jackie, that I had to go to work and leave her.'
> JC: 'Yes, because you went back to work when she was very young, didn't you?'
> 'She was a month old. My sister-in-law looked after her and that was the only thing I ever regretted. I don't think I was fair to her, but I had to go to work. If I wanted to dress her nicely and fed properly, then I had to go to work . . . She has had everything. It didn't matter what she ever asked for, what she wanted she got. I mean, even today, now she's married and got two children of her own, whatever she wants she has. Because I work and give it to her.'

Ann's sister and her brother-in-law frequently claimed that women's employment is the cause of all ills they see around them, but they did not mean to implicate either Ann or Betty, who also works, and Ann herself agreed with them. She resolved the apparent contradiction of working herself at the same time as condemning other women for working, by representing her own work as, simultaneously, vital to the family income and a comparatively unimportant 'little job'. The women whom she felt were at fault were women who want to work and who have 'real' jobs, i.e. jobs that are well-paid, and who treat their jobs in the same way as men:

> 'I think for a man, if his work is here, you've got to stay here. If his work's out and your work's here, it don't make no difference, you move out because you can always go and get a little job somewhere, it doesn't matter if the money's not a lot. But a man has to stay where his money is.'

Sarah Chalmers falls, as it were, between the generations. Too young to be middle-aged (she is in her mid-thirties), she is no longer a young mother. One of her children has already started work at the age of sixteen, and the other two are in secondary school. Sarah has had a succession of temporary jobs in the last ten years, but she has always been in work. Her husband, Mick, was in the room when she talked about her work in the interview, which made both of them uncomfortable. Sarah's wages are essential to the family income. She finds doing two jobs tiring and often wishes she could stop doing paid work, but there are aspects of going out to work she enjoys. Both she and Mick found the fact that she works and has to work difficult to integrate into the public account of the family that they wanted to give in the interviews, which involved Mick being the sole provider of the household:

> SC: 'I do prefer being at home. If I had, no, to be honest here, if you're single and you haven't got no housework to do, no cooking to do, no washing to do – I don't do no ironing because I hate it, the girls do it – then going to work is no problem. Because when you come home you haven't got to do nothing. But when you get up in the morning – this he classes as nagging – but when you get up in the morning and you do housework and you get the kids up and you get them ready and they go off to school and then you do a bit more housework and then you go off to work. You come back and then he comes back, and I make him a cup of tea and then I take the dog for a run, then I come back here. Then I sit down for an hour, then I go and make the dinner. It's on the go all the bloody time. And then he's got the cheek to turn round and say, "You don't do nothing of a night-time". I sit here and watch telly of a night. Didn't you?' (to Mick).
>
> MC: 'I agree with you. I don't think a woman should ever go out to work. I don't agree with it. I think a woman has enough work indoors. If you've got kids and you're running a home, I think that's enough for any woman.'

The main concern of the men and women of the middle generation in giving public accounts of their families, was to emphasize how well the family and the different members of the family functioned. There is a tradition of men being rough and occasionally violent which they find acceptable because it is not incompatible with the public account of a 'good father' and 'good husband' who is simply required to be hard-working, and occasionally to show 'who is boss' at home. To complement that image of men, the image of women in public accounts is one of their being steady, reliable, dependable, and accommodating. Ben Knight described his father as a one-time heavy drinker who gambled and got involved in fights but who later became teetotal and attended Church regularly. He made all these different aspects of his father's personality fit into the image of a 'good father':

> 'Our life was good. We never starved. He always worked and nothing was virtually too hard to do. And Christmas time, to bring up a family of that number. I can remember following him along to London Fields with a sack on me shoulder to buy, all right, it might not have been the best of fruit, but he used to always make sure we had the fruit and a gold penny in our socks, and an apple and some nuts. Never, ever turn round and say. Well, I say he was hard, but I think the hardness done me good in later life, because it made you really and truthfully respect, and I could see what I done wrong. Cause I was no saint, but the trouble is, I think to myself, that really and truthfully I would say that he held the family together.'

Because the man's role in the family is expected to be a minor one, the men in particular seemed to find it relatively easy to admit that the men in their own families were 'not saints', as Ben Knight put it, but they could not say the same of the women. Ben Knight's mother was 'a quiet, happy-go-lucky soul, and she always used to be smiling. Nothing was ever too much for her to do. And during her lifetime, I think she suffered a lot with my father.' The same contrast was apparent in Mick Chalmer's description of his grandparents with whom he lived until he was a teenager:

> 'Me grandfather was a bit of a sod, really, no-one liked him. Because me mother was from a family of nine, I think it was. Yes, nine in her family and me grandfather was a bit of a sod. They all hated him. He used to come home and beat them like they did in them days, he was a right drunkard and there wasn't a good word said about him. I got on all right with him, he gave me a few clouts mind you, but apart from that he was all right. And me Nan was as good as gold.'

It is noticeable, in Mick's reference to 'them days', which was also how Florrie Neagle talked about her parents, that behaviour that is not compatible with the respectability of public accounts can be talked about easily so long as it can be placed at a distance from the speaker. When people are talking about their close relatives or about relationships that exist in the present, there is a much higher premium on convention and acceptability, and a general insistence that domestic and family life works well. Asked about their husbands, the women say they are 'good husbands and good fathers'; asked about their wives, the men say they are 'good wives and good mothers'. Good husbands are hard workers and good fathers are men who make sure their children do not want for anything in the material sense. Good wives are good managers who handle the finances and do not make demands of their men and good mothers run the home and bring the children up well without too much difficulty. Mary Webb complimented her niece, Sharon, for 'having made a good job of her marriage' when no-one had expected her to, by which she meant that she had succeeded in turning her husband into a good husband and father when the rest of the family had thought he was an incorrigible tearaway. Joanne Goode said the main reason she left her first husband was because he would not go to work regularly and never managed to hold on to a job. Mick Chalmers said his reason for leaving his previous wife was that she had interfered in his leisure activities, she had not known her place.

For the younger people in the study the main features of the public account of family life are fundamentally the same, but there are minor differences. The first is that there was a vague commitment to a romantic view of marriage as a relationship between two people that both of them actively desires. The second is that there was an equally vague commitment to a less rigid sexual division of labour and to an idea that it is better for men to take a more active part in looking after their children. But these are only minor variations on the theme that family life works because it is based on a 'natural' sexual division of labour. William Cox described his father-in-law as going too far in expecting his wife to lay out his clean clothes and clean the bath after him, and said, 'I'm not as bad as that' (his wife denied this), but as the following quote shows, his view of the contractual nature of marriage was as traditional as his father-in-law's behaviour:

> 'When we was living at Stevenage, I seen a lot of marriages break up that was over money. Where they was going in the factories and bringing home, say, fifty pound a week wages and having to give their wife most of it. Most of the people up there was London people, where they'd been earning good wages, having a few bob to spend in the pub themselves. And what started happening? The husbands was holding the money back, the wives was having to scrimp and scrape, never going out, doing nothing, especially in the winter, 'cause the husband was

out drinking. To three of our friends it happened to. Or they was out of work and they was on each other's nerves, and they just broke up and it was all down to money. If they'd have had the money to do things, go out and have a nice home, giving their wives what they wanted to give them, it would never have happened.'

William's own approach to marriage and to his responsibilities towards his wife and children, apart from the fact that he referred to 'love', was no different from the traditional view that underlies all the public accounts of family life that have been examined:

'I love my work [he drives lorries]. I love her more than anything else. I'd stay at home, but I push her to the limit all the time. I stay out and do as much work as I know she'll stand. I go out at two o'clock in the morning and come home at ten at night because I know she'll stand for that. And if it meant me staying out all night, which I know she don't like and I don't like it myself, but I could do it. I could do it five nights a week, I could be away from home all week over work, but I give it to the others.'

In contrast with the public accounts of family life, which repeat the same images of men as good and hard-working and women as good and assiduously devoted to their families' welfare, so often that they begin to become predictable, the private accounts of family life in the interviews are idiosyncratic and unpredictable. They highlight the differences between individual men and women and the variety of personalities and relationships. The portrait that private accounts present of family life is chiefly characterized by stories of internal rifts within families, and of the stresses and strains individuals suffer because of their families and the various means they employ to overcome them. The examples of private accounts which are about to be presented have been selected from the interviews because they demonstrate, either by their content, or because they involve individuals whose public accounts have already been mentioned, the discrepancies between public and private accounts of family life.

The first concerns Mary Webb. At different times in her first interview Mary described her husband as variously, 'a marvellous father, he really is, the children have never wanted for anything, he's been a very loving father' and 'he's always been a very good worker'. Mary has eight children and, quite clearly, what she says is right: her husband does work extremely hard and provides a comfortable standard of living for nine other people besides himself. If this had been all she said, she would have successfully created the impression of a marriage that works well, and of a family that is basically untroubled and happy. But in the stories she told later, Mary revealed that her husband had refused to have anything at all to do with her every time she has been pregnant. With their last child, the period in which he had refused to talk to her had been prolonged for a further six months after the baby had been born. Mary described this aspect of her husband's behaviour as 'stupid', but she had also felt publicly humiliated by it because it was so much at odds with the image of a successful family which she felt it important to substantiate:

'He wouldn't talk to me, not until, he didn't even come to the hospital to see me when I had Ben [the last baby], he completely turned. And it was just in him. I suppose there are men like him who, I don't know, they turn like it, I suppose there is an explanation. But he would never explain it really. And I never asked him because I was very upset at the time. And I couldn't very well tell the sister in hospital that my husband was like a baby himself and refused to come and see me ... they put me in a side ward, which was just as well. I wanted to be on my own. And I had loads of visitors. In fact most of his family were so mad at him the way he turned out that they wouldn't even talk to him. But I had loads of visitors and I made out to the sister that my husband was working away at the time, you know, and he couldn't leave his job just to see me.'

Apart from her husband's 'stupid' reactions to her pregnancies, another of Mary's stories which did not fit her public account of her family, and which took some time (three interviews) to emerge, was about one of her daughters who, after having bitter verbal fights with both parents and being hit by her father, had left home. She had not gone far and was in fact living on the same estate as her parents, but if they met her, no-one in the family acknowledged her. In the interview, Mary whispered. 'We don't talk about her anymore'.

When Kathleen, Mary's sister, talked of her first marriage, she began by saying what a 'good husband and father' Harry had been. Mary, however, revealed that Harry had never been liked by Arthur Davies, partly because he had felt that it was bad for

Kathleen to be married to an invalid (Harry had suffered from tuberculosis before he met Kathleen and had it again in the course of their marriage), but mostly because Harry had treated Kathleen badly. In Mary's judgment, Kathleen was much better off with Stan Flowers:

'This other one Kathleen's got. I'm not being awful, but actually she looks much better since Harry died, to be honest with you, she never used to have two pennies to rub together. But now she's met Stan and she's definitely made a good recovery.'

Kathleen never mentioned being short of money as a problem in her first marriage, she was more concerned with the conflict between herself and Harry over the part he allowed his mother to play in their lives. It turned out that Harry had never taken her and the children out in the car at weekends without insisting that his mother accompany them. Kathleen disliked her mother-in-law and refused to go if she went. Harry had usually gone out with the children and his mother, and sometimes just with his mother on her own. The following passage in which Kathleen talks about Harry eventually coming to take her side against his mother is quoted for what it shows about the quality of the relationship that existed throughout most of their marriage:

'It was during that nine months' illness, that is when he turned against his own mother, sort of thing. Up until then it was always Mum and never me and the kids. But during that nine months, it doesn't matter what she'd done, she was wrong. And it was just me and the kids. And I said to my Mum, "Isn't it marvellous? The last nine months of our life had to be the happiest, really." Because you just couldn't do a thing wrong in the house, whatever you said, he went along with you. As soon as his mother opened her mouth, he used to bite her head off. And yet I'd been married to him for seventeen years and he'd never said "No" to her all that time. And it seems as if he had to be ill to make him see sense, you know, whose side he was on or who on his.'

There are other stories that reveal aspects of married life that people involved in the study either find unacceptable themselves or think others might find unacceptable: stories of husbands who are mean with their wages and do not give enough to their wives for the housekeeping; stories of husbands who refuse to go to work; of wives who nag and interfere in their husbands' leisure time; of mothers who are brutal to their children. The main impression created in private accounts is one of distance between husbands and wives, and often between parents and children, which is frequently, but not always, filled with bitterness and resentment. This is true even of the youngest of the married couples, the Coxes, with their vague commitment to a romantic ideal of marriage that the other couples do not share. Jackie Cox spends all day and the majority of evenings alone in the house with her three young children, and she is bored and frustrated. She would like her husband to spend more time at home and to help more with the housework: 'I would take more pride in the fact of saying that he helps me round my house because, after all, he lives in it as well.' In fact, William does nothing in the house and although this annoys her and leads to arguments between them, both of them see the house so much as her 'territory' that this is how she refers to it:

JC: 'You always talk about it as "my house". I've noticed that. And you talk about your Mum's house as "her house". As if your Dad . . . Do you know why that is?'
Jackie: 'I think it's cause I'm here all the time. I count it as my house. He says that to me actually. He says, "You say to me, 'Change my curtains'". He says, "They're not your curtains", and I say, "Well, they are really", 'cause he don't have a say. Well he does, but he says, "I might as well shut up".'

The private accounts of other relationships in families do not endorse the public accounts of families as harmoniously functioning units any more than the private accounts of marriages. This is especially true of the relationships between mothers and daughters which are the links between immediate and extended families. In public accounts, it is taken for granted that mothers and daughters help each other practically and that they do so willingly (and by implication happily) because 'blood is thicker than water'. The women in the Davies family seem to be an example of exactly this kind of relationship. Nellie helped her daughters in the past, and they help her in the present. Kathleen and Mary help their daughters in the present, and no doubt their daughters will help them in the future. All this is true, but it is at some cost to all of them, including Nellie. None of the daughters enjoy visiting their mother and often, because of this, are not as kind or as sympathetic as they might be. All of them find their obligations towards her tiresome and sometimes they seem unmanageable when there are other people in the family also making demands on their time. The help they give her is given resentfully rather than willingly, and because they feel that it is 'the right thing' to do.

In different ways, the public and private accounts of family life that we have examined in this section have all been concerned with the same thing: the way domestic life in these families is organized around a rigid and traditional sexual division of labour. In making the statement that family life works, and that it works *because* it is based on a 'natural' order of things, public accounts reproduce traditionalist ideology. In doing so, they legitimate the sexual division of labour as it stands in the study families, thereby ensuring both that women remain unequal in the labour market (and are thus easily exploited as cheap labour) and continue to supply the 'invisible' (because it is unpaid) domestic work that services their husbands and children (workers of the present and future) (Morpeth and Langton 1974; Gardner 1976; Frankenberg 1976). The private accounts do something different. They do not legitimate the sexual division of labour, but they do help people to accommodate to it more easily. The private accounts people gave of the more difficult or irritating or stressful aspects of family life were often given with a great deal of humour (see, for instance, the stories the women told about their husbands behaving 'like babies' when they are ill, reported in Chapter 5). In this instance, the service that they performed for the people who gave them was that they allowed them to laugh at the situation and, in doing so, get rid of 'bad' feelings. Private accounts tend to be given only when the person who is speaking is sure that what he or she is saying will be understood and accepted. Often the point of private accounts of family life seems to be to tell a story about an aspect of it that is not compatible with public accounts, precisely in order for the person telling the story to be able, in finding a sympathetic ear, to accept the reality of what they are talking about more easily.

There is very little hint of such aspects of family life in Young and Willmott's description of families in Bethnal Green, although much of what they had to say is replicated in the families involved in this study. Given the gap of almost thirty years that exists between the two studies, this is perhaps surprising. To take the most obvious of all the examples, there is apparently very little differrence between their description of 'matrifocal' families centred on the mother, and the case study of the Davies family reported in this chapter:

'The mother is the head and centre of the extended family, her home its meeting place. "Mum's is the family rendezvous" as one wife said. Her daughters congregate at the mother's house, visiting her more often than she visits any of them: 68% of married women last saw their mother at her home, and only 27% at their own. When there, they quite often see their other sisters, and brothers too, particularly if they are still living at home, but even if they live elsewhere, the sisters may call there at the usual time for a cup of tea, or just drop in for a chat on their way to the shops. Regular weekly meetings often supplement the day-to-day visiting.' (Young and Willmott 1957: 32)

However, the interpretation of family life in Bethnal Green in the two studies is very different, and the final section of the chapter to follow examines the reasons for this.

Family and kinship in East London: traditional working class solidarity?

The history of working-class family life, as Young and Willmott described it, had previously been a sorry one, and one for which men had largely been responsible:

'The husband too often took for himself what he should have spent on his family; an example, but a telling one, of his failure to co-operate with the person to whom God had joined him. . . . This was not the end of it. The husband was not only mean with money. He was callous in sex, as often as not forcing a trail of unwanted pregnancies upon his unwilling mate. . . . We cannot ignore the historical evidence, all the more so since the notion still survives that the working class man is a sort of absentee husband, sharing with his wife neither responsibility nor affection, partner only of the bed. Such a view is in the tradition of research into working class family life. The one aspect of that family which has been amply described is its failure.' (Young and Willmott 1957: 4–5)

But in their view, all this was now beginning to change, and a new 'partnership' between husband and wife was beginning to emerge; a partnership that would, incidentally, eventually succeed in undermining the matrifocal character of Bethnal Green families:

'The old style of working class family is fast disappearing. The husband portrayed by previous social investigation is no longer true to life. In place of the old comes a new kind of companionship between man and woman, reflecting the rise in status of the young wife and children which is one of the great transformations of our time. There is now a nearer approach to equality between the sexes and though each has a peculiar role, its boundaries are no longer so rigidly defined nor is it performed without consultation. The grand assumption made by Church and State (but thrown into doubt by earlier surveys) can be re-established ... men and women are partners.'
(Young and Willmott 1975: 15)

Their vision of an emerging partnership was based on evidence that fundamental changes had, or were, taking place in the pattern of working-class, and especially working-class men's existence. Men worked shorter hours than they had done previously and were free to spend more time at home with their families. Effective methods of contraception had produced a fall in the birth rate (which had in fact been particularly sharp in Bethnal Green (Gittins 1982)). Homes were less overcrowded than they had been, and the development of new, mass leisure activities such as the cinema and television, meant that men were choosing to spend more time with their families and at home, and less time in the pub, drinking. At the same time, and underlying these changes, working-class people's standard of living was rapidly improving, and husbands were beginning to make joint decisions with their wives about how to spend the family's income, and to form joint aspirations for their children.

To be fair to them, Young and Willmott were cautious about the extent of their claims ('We do not want to overdo it – these changes have not worked a revolution' (Young and Willmott 1957: 11)). Nevertheless, the evidence in this study suggests that their claims were exaggerated. The catalogue of social and economic changes which they presented has not brought about the fundamental change in relations between husbands and wives that they expected. On the contrary, the private accounts of domestic relations between men and women in this study are, if anything, closer to their description of the traditional view of the working-class family than they are to their own optimistic vision of a partnership between husbands and wives. Their expectation that the matrifocal character of family life would have changed and almost disappeared is also not borne out in the families involved in this study.

The problem with Young and Willmott's study is *theoretical*, insofar as their assumptions about the structure and meaning of family relationships made it difficult for them to interpret correctly what was going on in the families they studied, but it is also a problem of *research methods*. Their methods gave them access to public accounts of family life only, and they also made the fairly common mistake (see Mitchell 1969; Barnes 1969a; 1969b; Bott 1957; Harris 1969; Price 1981) of using quantitative measures to describe the quality of relationships, with misleading results for their interpretation of both marital and mother/daughter relationships.

Young and Willmott's analysis of the family is firmly based in the dominant paradigm of British sociology of the family, which is role theory (Morgan 1975). Role theory originates in Parsonian structural-functionalism, and Parsons's own application of the theory (Parsons and Fox 1968) is a sophisticated acknowledgment of the contradictory and stressful pressures of the family on its individual members. It is understood, for example, that men easily become scapegoats for things that go wrong in families because they have comparatively little to do with other family members, and that women have power in the home at the cost of being powerless outside it. In British sociology, role theory has been used in a much more ordinary and commonsense way in which the concept of role is understood as the social correlate of biological functions. Men have male roles outside the home; women have female domestic roles. The influence of role theory is evident in Young and Willmott's assumption that it is 'natural' for the relationship between the adult man and adult woman in a family to take precedence over other relationships, and that if it does not, this is something unusual, abnormal, and perhaps unnatural, and certainly in need of explanation.

In many of the families Young and Willmott studied in Bethnal Green, the women made it clear that they regarded their relationship with their mothers as more important than their relationship with their husbands and felt more attached to their mothers than to their husbands. Young and Willmott interpret this in two different ways. First, they suggest that the women's relationships with one another – which they call the women's 'trade union' – were a 'hang-over' from much worse social and economic conditions in the past which, once the standard of living began to improve, the women would be able to dispense with:

'These bonds, important still, probably counted even more in the earlier days of factory industry, when the mother-centred kinship system served to give working class women some security in a life beset by its opposite. The insecurity of men was translated into an even greater lack of security for women, who needed it more, then as always. In a district like Bethnal Green, wives could not rely upon their husbands to stand by them while they reared their children. Death too often removed the prop. Nor were they assured of support from husbands whose lives were spared. In an unstable economy, nearly all men were at some time unemployed and at all times frightened of it; and even when they were in work they frequently kept their families short of money. So the wife had to cling to the family into which she was born, and in particular to her mother as the only other means of assuring herself against isolation . . . The daughter's attachment to her mother is no longer such a compelling necessity now that the economy is more stable, broken homes fewer, the birth rate lower, and the husband's role in the family different.' (Young and Willmott 1957: 157–58, 159)

Second, they suggest that the women's relationships with their mothers were exclusive to the men and constituted an obstacle in the way of the married relationship developing:

'Mrs Warner, to instance another wife, was so identified with her mother that it turned out that when she said "us" during the interview she meant Mum and her, not her husband and herself. "We see so-and-so" meant "I see them at Mum's". Husbands so excluded from the feminine circle can be understood if they feel resentful of Mum's influence.' (Young and Willmott 1957: 47)

If the wife's mother is living near, the couple somehow have to adjust their lives to the fact that the wife is attached to her as well as to her husband. One course is for the husband to go his own way, spending a large part of his time away from his wife, not only during working hours, but at evenings and weekends as well. Another is for him to be drawn into the maternal fold along with his wife. In the past, we would suspect the second course was seldom followed, the pressures on the husband to exclude himself from the extended family, or be excluded, being too strong for most men to withstand.' (Young and Willmott 1957: 49).

Young and Willmott's concept of the 'right' relationship, meaning the relationship that is natural, normal, and proper – between mothers and daughters – was one that was principally based on their shared (biological) experience. They expected women to be emotionally close and personally supportive to one another, particularly around the physical and emotional aspects of becoming a mother, but without being interdependent:

> 'The daughter's attachment to her mother is no longer such a compelling necessity . . . but she still stands to gain a great deal from the person with whom she can share the mysteries, as well as the tribulations, the burdens, as well as the satisfactions of childbirth and motherhood . . . with a companion – and who more obvious for her to claim than the woman with whom she has shared her previous life?' (Young and Willmott 1957: 159)

The evidence from the families involved in this study does not support their interpretation on any of these three counts. First, the standard of living in Bethnal Green over the past thirty years has definitely improved but, judging by the case studies, relationships between mothers and daughters have changed very little. There is a great deal of sharing amongst the women, of housework and childcare. The basis for their relationships with one another is a mutual exchange of services principally, but not exclusively, services involving children.

Second, the women who took part in the study see each other apart from the men in their families, and at times when the men could not be affected by their visits to each other. Very occasionally, a husband accompanies his wife on a visit to her mother or sister, but usually in the company of the children so that the outing is a family event. For the most part, the women's relationships are conducted without the men even witnessing them. From Young and Willmott's account of the families they studied, the relationships between the women seem to have taken place on a similar basis: they saw each other mainly in the daytime when the men were at work, and the men were not much involved with their wives' families. This makes the idea of women 'excluding' men as the explanation of poor relations between husbands and wives somewhat unconvincing.

And third, whilst the relationships between the women are

based on a mutual exchange of services, the quality of their relationships is very varied. Some relationships are based on shared skills and practical activities and that is all; others involve some degree of emotional intimacy and the mother and daughter are each other's confidante; still others are based simply on family loyalty and a sense of duty. In some cases, of course, the relationship between a mother and her daughter involves all of these different dimensions – the relationship between Kathleen Read and her eldest daughter, Sharon, is a case in point – but the private accounts the women gave of their relationships made it clear that this was not always the case.

It is possible for there to be regular and frequent contact between mothers and daughters without either of them particularly liking the other, and even without any kind of practical interdependence. Kathleen, Joan, and Mary, for example, visit Nellie Davies regularly and provide her with all kinds of practical help and support but they resent her dependence on them and her lack of interest in their personal well-being. Jackie Cox and her mother, Ann, have a different type of relationship altogether. They see each other every day twice a day and once at weekends when they shop together, but Jackie never asks her mother for advice or help with the children because she does not regard her as qualified to give it. Ann did not look after Jackie when she was a child and as far as Jackie is concerned that means she knows nothing about children. If Jackie wants help or advice, she gets it from a friend her own age whom she sees as a 'real Mum'. The women in the study who expressed the most positive feelings about their mothers are not necessarily the most dependent on them for practical help, and the most dependent are not necessarily the most emotionally close. Joanne Goode, for example, Kathleen Read's second daughter, sees Kathleen every day twice a day and relies on her to look after her children and even for financial help in supporting them. But Joanne is not as close to her mother as her sister, Sharon, and never confides in her although, of the two of them, it is Sharon who is the least dependent.

There is no evidence either to support the idea that the natural form of the relationship between mothers and daughters is an intimacy and closeness that takes place around the 'mysteries' and 'tribulations' of pregnancy and childbirth. On the contrary, the women in the study were emphatic that they do not talk to their female relatives about such matters, and this is compatible with the evidence from another recent study in London which reports a 'real lack of knowledge about birth control and methods' amongst a group of young working-class women, 'in spite of the girls living close to their mothers' (Busfield 1974: 42). Nellie Davies, who in every other respect was a source of immense support and practical help to her daughters when they had their children, never, according to Kathleen, prepared them for the experience of childbirth:

'You had to find out all on your own. And the last words I can remember my Mum saying when I went into the ambulance were, "Well, when you go through it, just think 'Mum's been through it eleven times before'". I thought, "I wonder what the hell she means by that?" Of course, the flipping agony you go through, well, it's not agony really, it's fright and your not knowing what is happening.'

Young and Willmott's theoretical perspective on the family partially accounts for the exaggerated importance they attach to the partnership that was supposed to be emerging between husbands and wives and for their misunderstanding of the relationships between women. It ignores the necessary connection between women's biology and their 'trade unionism', which is their shared position in the sexual division of labour, and allows them to turn the relationships between women into an historical accident, the product of exceptionally poor material circumstances.

It is ironic that they should have chosen to draw an analogy between the relationships between the women and the trade unions because it is an analogy that is strikingly appropriate although not for the reasons they intended. By trade unionism, Young and Willmott meant that the women co-operate with each other in a mutually beneficial exchange of services, but the meaning can be pushed much further. Trade union organizations are built on the basis of shared positions in the system of production, but concern themselves mostly with their members' conditions of work and pay rather than with the much more fundamental question of control over the means of production. There is a parallel in the women's relationships which are based on a shared position in reproduction as well as in the system of production, but are actually more concerned with their conditions of work (helping each other out) than the much more fundamental question of control over their own fertility. It is understandable why the women should not discuss contraception, childbirth etc. together. Their structural position is such that they shoulder the entire burden of responsibility for the practical welfare of themselves and their children without having direct access to the material means to meet those responsibilities. Consequently, it is in their interest for relations between men and women to be subject to controls that ensure that they become regularized through joint domestic arrangements. The formal institution of marriage is less important than the fact that the men should meet their financial obligations towards the women and children.

One of the controls is over sexuality, which is the principal currency in which the exchange between men and women takes place. Sexuality and all subjects connected with it are partly controlled by making them taboo; they are either not talked about at all or they are talked about in restricted ways: laughter is one of the chief mechanisms that controls subjects related to sexuality in conversation. Contraception, pregnancy, and childbirth are all closely related to the matter of female sexuality and are therefore part of the taboo. Mothers do not discuss birth control with their daughters, but when their daughters get pregnant they put pressure on the man involved to marry them. There were signs in the interviews that this might be changing. Mary Webb's daughter, aged fifteen, became pregnant during the research period and Mary and her husband wanted her not to marry but to stay with them until she was allocated a flat of her own. Some of the younger women in the study said that they thought they would talk to their daughters about birth control and childbirth when they were older. If that happens, then it will be because they will have recognised that it is more obviously in their daughters' interests to know about these things because they will need to exercise control over their own fertility. Amongst other things, it is possible that this change in attitudes may be related to the single mother's entitlement to local authority housing which will move women one step away from total financial and material dependence on men and towards greater independence.

There are also methodological reasons for why Young and Willmott should have misinterpreted family life and relationships. *Family and Kinship* is based partly on a period of observation in Bethnal Green and partly on two types of interviews: a standard survey-type of interview which they describe as 'formal and standardised, the questions being precise and factual, with a limited range of alternative answers', and a relatively 'intensive' interview with a smaller sample of forty-five married couples (Young and Willmott 1957). They had wanted to interview husbands and wives separately but in the majority of cases found this impossible to arrange. However, they did manage to see half the wives on their own in the daytime.

On the face of it there is very little difference between Young and Willmott's method of interviewing the married couples and the interviews undertaken for this study, but the two approaches are fundamentally different. Young and Willmott's Schedules for Intensive Interviews concentrate on formal arrangements – on who people see regularly, how much time they spend together, where they meet, and so on. The interviews for this study concentrate on the reasons people have for seeing each other and how they feel about their relationships. Young and Willmott assumed, wrongly, that the formal properties of relationships are a valid indicator of their content and quality. In the case of married couples, this means that they chose, for example, to use the number of times husbands did the washing-up in a week as an index of their participation in and contribution to domestic work, and the amount of time they spent at home as an indicator of their involvement in the family. McKee points out (1982: 123) that quantitative measures of this kind ignore the key domestic issues of who has overall responsibility for the running of the house, who knows what needs to be done, who has the forethought and makes the plans that are necessary if the next meal is to appear on the table, if everyone is to have clean clothes and essential supplies are not going to run out. We also know from the case studies that the amount of time a man spends at home is meaningless in itself. We need to know what he does whilst he is at home because if he spends most of the time asleep or in front of the television, his involvement in the family can remain minimal. Equally, as has already been pointed out, if mothers and daughters see each other regularly, this does not necessarily mean they are personally and emotionally close.

In the majority of cases, Young and Willmott interviewed husbands and wives together, and it is worth considering that this makes it more rather than less likely that the people they interviewed gave public accounts of their families, or 'morally correct answers', as Morgan calls them (1975). Public accounts of family life in the interviews are perfectly compatible with role theory and it is not difficult to see how from within that theoretical perspective it could be assumed that, for example, if a woman says that she is close to her mother and there is nothing they do not talk about together, it means that they talk about pregnancy, childbirth, etc. The analysis of the interviews in this study shows that the reality is more complicated. In a public account a woman can say quite truthfully that she talks to her mother about everything without denying the (privately admissible) fact that there are certain things they never talk about.

Conclusion

This critique of Young and Willmott's work has come full circle, to end back at the point where it started, that of the different aspects of family life portrayed in public as opposed to private accounts. This is an important point because so much of our understanding depends on our theoretical approach to the way in which people discuss their own lives.

This chapter is part of the attempt to construct a framework within which the much more explicit discussion of health and illness and health services in the next three chapters can take place. The character of the domestic division of labour and its legitimations in the study families are integral to that framework. For example, it will be relevant to know that the responsibility for housework and childcare is entirely borne by women who treat this as their job and that this carries all the moral significances of work examined in Chapter 3; that in practice, 'parental' responsibility means 'maternal' responsibility, especially as far as the child's physical well-being is concerned; and that the subjects one might expect to be talked about in families and between women are not in fact discussed, so that relatives are not necessarily a source of health information. Finally, the tentative connections that have been made in this chapter between attitudes towards birth control and women's structural position suggests the importance of analysing health matters generally in the context of people's lives as a whole.

5 Concepts of Health and Illness

The point has now been reached where the description of the people and of their way of life is complete, and discussion of their relationship to health and illness and to doctors and the health service has not yet begun. The purpose of this chapter is to form a link showing the relevance of preceding chapters for understanding the interview material concerned with health and illness. The concept of 'medicalization' is used to explain the relationship that people in the study have not only with medicine (both as a science and as a clinical practice), but with matters of health more generally.

The concepts of medicalization and 'the medicalization of life' are well known in medical sociology. This study disagrees with the interpretation of medicalization in the 'medicalization of life' thesis and these disagreements are outlined in the first section of this chapter. However, it has retained the concept of 'medicalization' because it is valuable. 'Medicalization' implies *relationship*, and it implies *interaction between* two worlds (Habermas calls them 'systems of action' (Habermas 1971)) which are different and separate from each other. One is the world of lay people and of commonsense health beliefs; the other is the world of medicine and of applied science. 'Medicalization' further implies that the relationship between the two is not equal and that it is dominated by medicine. The acknowledgement that two parties are involved and that there is an unequal process of interaction between them provides a framework that is appropriate to the analysis of the discussions about health and illness and about health services that took place in the interviews.

This is the first of three chapters that deal directly with the topics of health and illness. It aims to establish the meaning of 'medicalization' as it is used in the study, and to show the relevance of the concept for the analysis of the meanings of health and illness contained in the interviews. Chapters 6 and 7 to follow apply the concept of medicalization to the analysis of the aetiological theories that people put forward in their interviews and to the relationship that people in the study have with doctors and with different sections of the health service.

As in previous chapters, the interview material is presented in two sections, one that is concerned with the meaning of health and illness in public accounts, and one that is concerned with the meanings in private accounts. As before, the distinction between the two types of account is partly based on the – now familiar – distinction between people answering 'public' or apparently formal questions ('What was/is your mother's/father's/children's health like?', 'How is your own health?'), and people telling stories about their own or other people's personal experience. It is also always possible to characterize public accounts in terms of their overriding preoccupation with questions of acceptability and legitimacy. This is as true of public accounts of health and illness as it is of public accounts of other matters, only in this instance, because the topic concerns health, the issue is complicated by the fact that there is a public hierarchy of authorities in relation to health matters which is topped by medicine. This means that public accounts of health and illness not only have to be acceptable to the 'public' (as represented by the other person), but that the people who are giving them also have to be concerned about their legitimacy with respect to medicine. However, to complicate matters further, the difference between public and private accounts of health does not simply correspond to a difference between medical and lay concepts. It is not, to use the terminology of the medical anthropologists (Eisenberg 1977; Helman 1978), a matter of public accounts reproducing medical concepts of *disease* whilst private accounts produce lay concepts of *illness*. Public accounts contain both medical and lay concepts, and switch between them, depending on the form of legitimation which is most applicable to the subject and the context in which it is being discussed at any particular moment. Moreover, in both types of account, professional medicine is the final authority which establishes whether a particular event or occurrence concerning the health of a person will be considered 'real', and therefore legitimate, or 'not real' and therefore illegitimate.

These points are developed and clarified in the discussion that follows. The chapter is divided into three sections: the first defines 'medicalization' and describes the main differences of interpretation with the 'medicalization of life' thesis; the second and third sections apply the concept of medicalization to the analysis of the meanings of health and illness in public and in private accounts.

The concept of medicalization

This study takes medicalization as one instance of the much broader process of 'rationalization' which Habermas defines as the key process in modernization (Habermas 1971). All social systems have their own forms of legitimation – Habermas calls them 'action-orienting' and 'power-legitimating' traditions – which provide the explanations, the reasons, and the justifications for people's actions and for social relationships. According to Habermas, all such traditions are 'ideological' in the sense that they 'keep actual power relations inaccessible to analysis and to public consciousness' (Habermas 1971: 99). This is not to say that the public consciousness is 'false' and that people are misled or that they are duped into believing untruths, but to imply that the deep structures underlying social action and social relations are hidden, are not self-evident, and are not revealed by the various legitimating traditions associated with them. Habermas distinguishes between two types of legitimations or legitimating procedures: traditional legitimations which are 'normative', i.e., they involve questions of human values and are associated with religious, metaphysical, or moral systems of belief; and modern legitimations which are scientific and technical and are derived from analytic or empirical knowledge. 'Rationalization' is the process that takes place when social life is transformed by traditional legitimations being overturned and replaced by modern ones.

The process of rationalization takes place on two levels, the level of culture as a whole (rationalization 'from above'), and the level of sub-cultures and individuals (rationalization 'from below') (Habermas 1971: 96–9). At both levels, the process is the same: traditional legitimations are undermined and they lose their cogency – people lose faith in them – in the face of modern scientific and technical forms of argument which eventually replace them. Medicalization as used in this study is the specific form which rationalization takes in the area of health and illness. Medicalization 'from above' describes the changes in the Western view of mind and body that have occurred with the development of scientific medicine. Medicalization 'from below' describes the changes in social life and social relations that create a readiness on the part of sub-cultures and the individuals who belong to them to accept modern (in this case, medical) legitimations for health and illness where once they accepted traditional (commonsense and moralistic) legitimations. It also refers to the impact the practical achievements of scientific medicine make on the collective consciousness.

The advantage of using this conception of medicalization in the analysis of the interview material lies in the acknowledgement that the relationship of lay people to medicine, and thus, by extension, to matters of health and illness generally, can be analysed on different levels. It states the dominant tendency in our culture, which is towards modern scientific and technical forms of legitimation, without implying that the process will necessarily be carried through everywhere and in all social groups, at the same pace or at the same time. The rate of progress of medicalization depends upon the state of readiness of sub-cultures and of individuals within sub-cultures to allow it to take place, and on their state of awareness and knowledge of scientific achievements.

The differences between this definition of medicalization and the interpretation of medicalization in the 'medicalization of life' thesis, can be summarized under four headings. These have been adapted from Strong's (1979a) ten-point summary of the assumptions underlying the 'medicalization of life' thesis, or the notion, as he put it, of 'medical imperialism'.

1) *The medical profession*: the 'medicalization of life' thesis represents 'medicine' and 'the medical profession' and 'the medical establishment' as unitary phenomena. It ignores the institutional divisions within medicine and the conflicts and disagreements that exist between doctors and groups of doctors, between specialist groups and between the different branches of the profession. This is rightly described by Strong as crude over-simplification (1979a). This study does not support a unitary conception of medicine. It attempts, where possible, to meet Strong's point, and to specify the differences and divisions amongst doctors and within the health service in East London, as they affect the empirical material and the analysis of the empirical material. However, in the discussions that follow, it is often necessary to distinguish between the 'medical' and the 'lay', as for example in the difference between medical and lay concepts, or medical and lay theories of aetiology, and it is difficult to do so without seeming to support either a unitary conception of

medicine or the idea (also much criticized by Strong) of *a* medical model. It should therefore be made clear that when the term 'medical' is used, the reference is to *dominant* sections within the profession and to *dominant* concepts of health/illness in medicine. There are hierarchies in medicine and they are involved in the creation of medical orthodoxy; there are also theories and forms of practice which at any one time will be more popular and more common amongst doctors than other alternatives, and it is these that represent medical orthodoxy. The section (or sections) and view (or views) that dominates is usually associated with the medical schools and with acute hospital medicine rather than with general practice, chronic care, or preventive medicine. It is these that will be meant by the use of the term 'medical' in this chapter and the chapters to follow.

2) *Ideology*: the 'medicalization of life' thesis defines medicine as an institution of social control, and the control it exercises as 'ideological'. The term 'ideology' is interpreted in various different ways, all of which treat the links between medicine and social/political control of populations as more obvious and more direct than Habermas's definition of 'ideology' (see, for example, Zola 1978; Navarro 1977). This study defines medicine as ideological in the sense of Habermas referring to the legitimating functions of science and technology when he says that all legitimations are ideological because they keep 'actual power relations inaccessible to analysis and to public consciousness'. (Figlio's study (1978) of the nineteenth century concept of 'chlorosis' uses historical material to make the same point.) It argues also that the fact that medicine is an *applied* science is significant. Medicine is, in a sense, the most human of science's faces and, as such, it plays a key role in establishing the status and authority of science and technology as sources of legitimation in modern society.

3) *Medical imperialism*, and 4) *Patients*: the 'medicalization of life' thesis defines medicine as a 'radical monopoly' (Illich 1976) which is continually annexing to itself areas of 'ordinary life' previously under moral, religious, or legal jurisdiction (Zola 1978). The way it supposedly does this is by destroying 'traditional health care resources' in communities so that the individuals belonging to these communities are forced to transfer their dependence away from these traditional supports and on to medicine and the medical profession. The relationship between 'the medical profession' on the one side and 'patients' on the other, is portrayed as a one-sided affair in which patients have

given themselves over uncritically and without question to medical control. Having become dependent on medicine, people are said to become 'addicts', wanting more attention, more medication, more intervention, and so on.

The argument does not take account of historical or anthropological evidence concerning medical practice in our own society in the past or in societies other than our own, and is not supported by current empirical studies of patients' attitudes and behaviours (Strong 1979a). The data which are available show class and other social differentials in patients' use of health services which indicate that the 'addiction' these authors are afraid of, if it exists at all, is restricted to a tiny proportion of the population (Townsend 1974; Tudor Hart 1971; Townsend and Davidson 1982). The same data show differentials in the use of different types of services, with the services that are most clearly in line with the medicalization of life argument – i.e. the preventive and screening services which attempt to treat non-sick people – being the most under-used. Far from being addicts of medicine, these studies show that most patients attempt to treat their own illness before consulting a doctor, make infrequent use of the health service, and are critical of the services that are available to them (Cartwright 1967; Stimson and Webb 1975; Strong 1979a).

The evidence in the interviews for this study does not support the interpretation of medicalization in the 'medicalization of life' thesis, but matches Habermas's discussion of rationalization/medicalization perfectly. The interviews show that medical and lay concepts of health and illness are related, that the relationship is not equal, and that the medical view dominates. There are also some indications in the interviews that innovations in medical science and clinical practice affect lay health beliefs (see for example the discussion of changing attitudes towards the menopause as a result of hormone replacement therapy – (pp. 132–33). There is no evidence to support the idea that medicine's jurisdiction has extended or has been accepted in areas not considered 'properly' medical, i.e. relevant to physical and mental health, whilst there is some evidence to suggest that even in conventionally 'medical' areas such as ante-natal and obstetric care and infant and child health, its jurisdiction is contested (see pp. 190–96).

The outcome of the process of rationalization, as Habermas describes it, is an 'urbanized form of life' (Habermas 1971: 98) in which people learn to 'switch between' one action-orienting tradition and another. In the context of this discussion, this means that people are capable of 'switching between' a traditional (in this case a moral or commonsense) approach to health and one that is modern (in this case medical and scientific). This notion of individuals and sub-cultures having both traditional (normative) and modern (scientific) legitimations to draw upon, and switching between the two, is substantiated by the discussions about health and illness which took place in the interviews.

The sections of this chapter that follow demonstrate the relevance of the concept of medicalization for the interpretation of the content of both public and private accounts of health and illness as well as for the interpretation of the discrepancies between the two types of account. In the interviews, people did switch between commonsense concepts of health and illness which had obvious connections with their moral philosophy, and medical concepts or concepts they believed to be medical in origin. They also put forward commonsense explanations of health and illness that incorporated medical concepts and theories. Here it was less a matter of 'switching between' the two 'systems of action' than of their own commonsense beliefs 'reflecting and embodying the perspectives developed by experts' (to paraphrase Giddens (1976: 115)). At another level also, much of the content of discussions about health and illness – including the use of medical terms – can only be properly understood in the context of their lives as a whole. The private accounts in particular show that the relationship people in the study have with health matters of all kinds is powerfully moulded by the practical constraints of work and family life which dominate their lives and by the meanings these constraints hold for them.

Public accounts of health and illness

The public accounts of their own health and of their relatives' health histories which people gave in their interviews were couched in commonsense terms from which it was clear that health and illness are considered morally problematic conditions. The exact meanings of both terms, as people used them, was never taken for granted but was always 'negotiated' by the person giving the account. The person always made sure that they were seen to be in the 'right', i.e. the morally correct position in relation to them. The 'right' relationship to these terms was that of being basically healthy; if illnesses were mentioned, people made sure that they were understood to be 'real' and therefore legitimate.

The very first indication of the problematic nature of the topics of health and illness came right at the beginning of the study when people were being approached to take part in the interviews. Sometimes they had already agreed to be interviewed before they had properly grasped the fact that they would be asked to talk about their health, at which point they changed their minds and tried to back out; sometimes they refused, insisting that there was 'no need' for them to be included in the study because their health and their children's health was good, and it would be better to ask someone else – perhaps an old person – who could tell me more than they could. The assumption was always that a 'health study' was an 'illness study', and they wanted no part of it. When these same people were eventually persuaded that they should be interviewed, it was on the understanding that this was a study of health and illness in 'ordinary people' and that they had not been selected and would not be presented as people with particularly acute health problems.

The initial statements which people made about how good their health was bore no relation to their medical histories. When she was first contacted, Mary Webb made the usual disclaimers about being part of the study because she had 'never been ill in her life', although she acknowledged that she had been in a motorbike accident in her teens and had spent two months in hospital after it. Later, when she was interviewed, it emerged that Mary had had a number of episodes of acute illness in the past ten years (the most serious an acute form of anaemia which had required emergency hospital treatment and many blood transfusions) but she had also had measles immediately after the birth of her fourth child (in six years), which had made her very ill, and a kidney infection for which she had out-patient treatment for two years. Mary's sister, Kathleen, was another person who described herself as 'healthy': Kathleen, in fact, had said when we first met that she was 'lucky' to have such good health. Kathleen's medical history included having had such bad eyesight as a child that she was expected to be blind by the age of twenty, lung disease including tuberculosis in her late teens, a miscarriage, a thyroid deficiency which requires permanent medication, and, six years prior to the interviews, a hysterectomy. Confronted with the contradiction between her initial claim that she had never been ill and the facts of her medical history, Mary explained that she did not like to see herself or to be seen by anyone else as someone with poor health, and that she particularly disliked talking about her health because she was worried that she would be mistaken for a 'moaner'. Kathleen's only comment about the matter was: 'If you can't go through life without bearing a little bit of pain, you might as well die.'

Mary and Kathleen's mother, Nellie Davies, was generally characterized by everyone in the family as a 'moaner', and, as such, she embodied everything that her daughters and everyone else who was interviewed wanted not to be associated with. She was, in fact, the only person who was interviewed and the only close relative who was talked about in this way. No-one in Nellie's family mentioned her name without complaining about the fuss she made about her health, and whilst recognising that she did have specific health problems, they were not sympathetic towards her method of coping with them:

KR: 'You know she's not lying, but it's no good keep moaning because we can't do nothing. She's had the doctor in and all he's done is given her circulation tablets. And they're, her poor legs, the skin is so bad on them, he's not even given her a bit of cream for them. To me that's bad, to be honest. I think, well, she's got a right to moan now because she's brought him home when she can't get out to see him and yet he's given her nothing. So, in a sense, she has got a reason for moaning as far as she's concerned but then it's no good moaning to us because we can't do nothing about it anyway. It's no good us going to him and saying we demand this and demand that, because you're not going to get it anyway.'

JC: 'Do you think it makes it more difficult to tell how he is?

KR: 'Well, I think it does really. Because, all right, she takes her heart tablets, she's making it worse on herself by moaning, to be honest. And I know her hands are bending over because her hands are so cold she's got no feeling in them, but there again, she could have seen that they were seen to before she got as bad as they are now.'

KR: 'I think she does actually try to see if you're going to feel sorry for her, to be honest. But she's pushed us all too far and you can't feel sorry for her any more, to be honest. Just turn round and say, "How she is now is what she's brought on herself".'

MW: 'It seems Mum must be the, everyone must fall over themselves to ask Mum how she is, and Mum must be the one you ask. No use asking Mum, "How's Dad?". She doesn't want to know about it, it's how she is. When she starts looking at her hands and rubbing her hands and saying "I can't feel my hands, they've gone so cold", well, she's had this trouble for donkey's years, but it's just one of those things, because the blood's not going to her heart like it used to and it's just old-age problems. And we know it can be dangerous when she picks up a hot kettle and she could drop it and things like that. She's had one or two very nasty burns. And she still dwells on things so much. It's always how ill she is and if she phones you up it's not, "Hello Mary, how are you?". Straight away it's "I feel so awful and ill" and things like that. And if one day she does ask you how you feel, I think you'd pass out with shock.'

The interview with Nellie bore out her relatives' descriptions of her behaviour. She did complain about her hands being cold, about having internal pains and about being neglected by the doctor. She also looked as if she had a great deal to complain about. She was extremely thin and frail and her hands and legs, and apparently most parts of her body including the inside of her mouth, were affected by sores that were open and infected.

The comments about Nellie have been quoted at some length because, along with other more random comments about particular individuals – usually acquaintances or neighbours – who were thought to be overly preoccupied with their health, they shed some light on why people had not wanted to take part in a 'health study' and why they insisted that their health was good. There was general agreement amongst people in the study that certain *other* people were hypochondriacs. These were people who were never 'really' ill, who fussed too much about minor health problems that were not 'proper' illnesses, and who enjoyed poor health because they had 'nothing better to do with their time' than go to the doctor's. Many people enjoyed telling stories about hypochondriacs which proved that they were not ill at all. One of these was a story about Stan Flowers' sister-in-law, a woman who had always insisted that she was too much of an invalid to do her own housework and whose husband had done it for her, but who, when he died, had made a remarkable recovery and had started going out drinking every night and generally enjoying herself. In a different vein altogether, stories were also told about other people, the very opposite of hypochrondriacs, who were held up as objects of respect and of admiration. Kathleen remembered a fellow-patient in the sanatorium, an ex-nurse with tuberculosis in her joints who, despite being in great pain and knowing that her career was ended, was always happy and cheerful. Joe Hutchinson was enormously proud of the fact that no-one had known how ill his wife had been in the last few years of her life because she had always managed to give the impression of being so well, and Jeannie Moss had had an aunt whom she remembered with great affection, who had managed to conceal from all but her closest relatives that she had tuberculosis.

From the stories of hypochondriacs and stoics, it was clear that people in the study had not wanted to be interviewed about their health in case it should be assumed that they too enjoyed illness as a topic of conversation. Their initial refusals to take part in the study sprang from an anxiety that to talk about health – meaning illness as they understood it – might be to take the risk of being considered a hypochrondriac. Even after they had agreed to be interviewed, some people continued to feel uneasy about what they were doing, and in it least one case, this led to the person leaving their most serious illness out of their medical history, a fact which came to light much later, over an informal cup of tea, without the tape recorder running.

Underlying the content of public accounts of health, which can be characterized as commonsense legitimations – the insistence on one's own health being good, the scorn for hypochrondriacs, the proofs of the 'reality' of illness and resistance to it – lies a set of moral philosophical reflections on the nature of health and illness which replicate exactly the reflections on work and the nature of individuals' responsibility for their work, considered in Chapter 3. There are obvious reasons why work and health should be connected in people's minds. Illness can incapacitate and prevent people from working. In doing so, it can threaten not only the practical basis of their lives but also their moral reputation (see Chapter 3). The moral philosophical argument which connects the two is less obvious, but it is nonetheless fundamental to the recurrent theme in public accounts of health and illness of 'good health' being a morally worthy state, and illness being discreditable.

The public accounts of both health and work argue that inequality is a product of nature, but at the same time they hold individuals responsible for their place in the hierarchy. The interviews contain many statements to the effect that health is 'a lottery', a matter of luck, fate, or destiny, because whether or not one is healthy depends on whether or not one was *naturally* endowed with a good '*constitution*'. 'The things you have wrong with you, you're normally born with', as William Cox put it. (The statement has obvious parallels with the idea that natural differences (inequalities) of intelligence and ability explain occupational and social hierarchies.) However, good health is also said to be the reward for a good life, meaning a life of moderation and virtue, cleanliness and decency, and above all, a life of hard work. In other words, just as one's place in the hierarchy has to be achieved by 'making the most of oneself', so too one's health has to be 'earned'.

Although most people in the study were at pains to point out that they were not religious, by which they meant that they were not regular church-goers, they based their belief in the possibility that good health could be 'earned' on the notion of a morally just God. When events ran contrary to the scenario of moral investments and just rewards, they expressed a bitterness about life that was a bitterness in the fact of an unjust God. Joan Young, for example, could not accept that her father 'deserved' to lose a leg, because he had always been a 'good husband' and a 'good father', and he had always worked hard. She prefaced her comments on his operation by saying, 'They say there is a God above, but I doubt it'. Betty Mayes was equally at a loss to explain how her brother and two sisters could have had cancer:

'They've all worked. I mean, my sister who's sixty-odd now, she retired when she was sixty, she's always worked. We've all worked. My eldest sister who died, she had all her own business. She sold her business up and bought a house at Romford. They went in the middle of December. She was dead in May. She worked all her life. My other sister who died, she worked right up.'

And her sister, Ann, had the same sense of injustice talking about these illnesses:

'I don't know. I can't understand any of it really. I know when my brother first died – I used to work in Aldgate then – and I used to go to work and see the old methers lying in the road drunk and all that. And I used to think to myself, "Why? My brother had to die at fifty. A hard-working man, had a good wife and a nice home." Yet if you see them. I know I shouldn't say it, if like I realised afterwards, I thought, "I'm being wicked".

Because it doesn't matter who you are or how you live, life's still sweet. But sometimes it do make you feel a little bit bitter when you know your own have worked so hard and led a good life, and then you see all that. And you think to yourself, "Why?". I don't know, but I suppose that's how it's meant to be.'

As we have seen in Chapter 3, the people involved in this study do not have much control over their working lives and yet they take upon themselves the injunction to work hard and make the most of themselves regardless of the nature of the work they are doing. There is a direct parallel in the attitude they adopt towards their health. They experience themselves as having very little control over whether or not they are healthy and yet they take seriously the idea that having the 'right attitude' is the passport, if not to good health, at least to a life that is tolerable. The moral prescription for a healthy life is in fact a kind of cheerful stoicism, evident in the refusal to worry, or to complain, or to be morbid. Taking an interest in health is itself regarded as morbid. Stan Flowers looked appalled when I asked if he ever discussed his health or anything to do with health with his friends at the local working-men's club, and said that men who did so were ostracized for being morbid. Sharon Berthot illustrated the point with this story about her husband's cousin whom she considered a 'crank' and a 'health fanatic':

'He sort of went berserk and he took an overdose because he couldn't, what was it? He couldn't bear the thought of bringing up his children in this sort of world. Disease and things like that. He went, he flipped his lid, he went completely potty because. If you went round you wasn't allowed to smoke in the room where the children were, he wouldn't drink, and he went onto one of those, a fresh food thing, only fresh food, no tinned stuff, no preservative and all. All I mean he ended up in St Clements, he went off his rocker. I thought, if that's what worrying does to you, what's the point of worrying?'

In the course of the interviews, it was of course impossible for people to avoid mentioning illness altogether, and once a particular illness had come to light in this context the onus on the person giving the account was that of proving that the illness was 'real' and that it was therefore legitimate for them – or whoever was involved – to be a patient. The basic requirement was that they should be able to prove the 'otherness' of the illness, i.e., prove that it was a recognisable and separate entity which had 'happened' to the person and not something for which they were personally responsible. It is at this point that the interaction between commonsense and medical legitimations which characterizes the medicalization process can be identified. The most conclusive proof of the 'reality' of an illness the person could offer was a medical diagnosis. The scientific discourse of medicine thus provided the major solution to the moral difficulties of illness; once there was a recognisably medical diagnosis the questions of individual responsibility and culpability were no longer relevant. Lesser proofs of the 'reality' of illness involved showing one had nothing to do with causing it, that the symptoms were tangible and obvious, and that the illness was incapacitating – one had neither 'given in' to it, nor 'given up'.

Certain categories of health problem were not problematic in the sense that it was not difficult for people to admit to having had them. These were accidents and illnesses whose 'otherness' could be taken for granted. The category of illness which was recognisably medical can be broken down into 'normal' illness and 'real' illness. The former describes commonplace illness which medicine treats and treats successfully; the latter describes illness that is unusual or severe and which is as yet either just within or just beyond the province of successful medical treatment. The category people had the most difficulty with was the category that we call 'health problems that are *not* illness'. These are problems which medicine does not treat or for which the treatments that are available are only partially successful. They are also problems which are thought in some way to be connected to the person who has them, either through their personality, their age, or their way of life; problems whose 'otherness' cannot be taken for granted.

The following tri-partite classification indicates the range of health problems included in each of the three categories:

(i) 'normal' illness: the model for 'normal' illness is the infectious diseases which children are expected to catch – chickenpox, mumps, measles, and rubella. The definition includes some illnesses of childhood that medicine has relegated to the past – e.g., whooping cough and scarlet fever – and infectious illness in adults that is not severe. Infections of the kidneys, tonsils, sinus, stomach, and boils and abcesses are all included, as well as fever and 'flus and some common respiratory diseases.

(ii) 'real' illness: the model for 'real' illness is established by the major and 'modern' disabling and life-threatening diseases, i.e., cancers and cardiovascular and coronary heart diseases. The 'reality' of the illness is established by the poor prognosis and by the impact it makes on the patient. Epilepsy, diabetes, and other chronically disabling illnesses which require constant medication are included. 'Real' illness definitely falls within the province of medicine but that is not to say that all illness in this category is treatable. The definition refers to the severity and therefore to the 'stature' of the condition rather than to whether or not medical help actually exists or is successful.

(iii) 'health problems which are not illness': these are problems associated with natural processes – of aging and of the reproductive cycle – and problems that are thought to stem from the person's nature or personality, such as allergies, asthma, and eczema. The common feature of this category of problems is that they are thought not to be amenable to medical treatment. Sometimes some form of self-treatment may be advocated. Health problems that are regarded as a natural part of growing old are: rheumatism, arthritis, digestive disorders, varicose veins, palpitations, and feeling the cold, as well as loss of hearing and vision. The problems that menstruation and the menopause account for are many and various: they include abdominal pain, sickness, nausea, palpitations, hot flushes, blood loss, changes in weight, faintness and dizziness, depression and other mood changes, and changes in the condition and texture of skin and hair.

If the legitimacy of the illness can be established, the moral implications of having it fall away. The key point is that by establishing the 'otherness' of the illness the person is able to prove that they are not personally responsible for it because it is something that falls within (and comes from) the province of medicine. The onus of doing the right thing is still on them, but it becomes a question of taking appropriate action rather than seeking to prove either that one is not ill at all, or, if the illness is manifestly obvious, has not caused it.

If the person is unable to establish the legitimacy of his/her condition, i.e., if the problem is defined as a 'health problem that is not illness', then the moral status of the condition itself remains problematic and the effort to prove that one is not responsible is that much greater. People were much more careful to put themselves in the 'right' relation to illnesses in the third category than they were with the other two categories. The following examples illustrate the point. The first concerns an instance in which Daniel Mayes had mentioned in passing that his nephew had eczema as a child before catching it himself, and he went back to the topic in an effort to prove that this was not something for which either the nephew or his parents were to blame:

> 'It's a disease, isn't it? And I don't think they really know how it occurs or anything like that. And it's definitely not through dirt because, as Bet will tell you, my sister's house is as clean if not cleaner than most people's. Hygenic, you know. And it wasn't through the food because her cooking, she's a real good cook so it's not through neglect, not eating bad foods or tinned foods.'

The key phrases in this passage are, 'It's a disease', and 'I don't think they really know how it occurs'. Anything that is recognised by medicine can be classified as a 'disease', meaning something 'other', and as long as 'they don't know what causes it', it cannot be proved that the person is responsible.

The other example concerns the menopause and hormone replacement therapy. The most common attitude towards the menopause amongst the women who were interviewed was that it was natural for women to have difficulties with their health when they were going through 'the change', but that the 'right' approach was to put up with these difficulties without fussing about them, and certainly without bothering the doctor. However, they also knew that medical treatment – hormone replacement therapy – was available to treat the discomfort and unpleasant symptoms that sometimes accompany the menopause, and the implications of such a treatment existing at all were that they might not have to accept these symptoms as 'natural' and 'inevitable' and as 'not illness' but 'part of the reproductive cycle'. As yet, this had not happened; the menopause was in a transitional position with some women choosing to seek medical help and others maintaining a more traditional approach.

The confusion around the moral/medical status of menopausal symptoms had caused some conflict between women who were involved in the study. At the time of their interviews, both Carol McInnes and her friend, Jeannie Moss, were going through the menopause. Jeannie had had hot flushes but very little else, whilst Carol had been depressed and had many other complaints and symptoms. Carol was taking hormone treatments and insisting that she needed them because she was unable to cope without them, whereas Jeannie's attitude was that she was making an unwarranted fuss. This was something that happened to all women, and she saw no reason for Carol to think that it was worse for her than it was for anyone else.

In their public accounts of health and illness, the people who were interviewed were mainly preoccupied with moral aspects of health and illness. They perceive health and illness as matters that are largely beyond the powers of the individual, dictated by natural inequalities in the basic constitutional make-up of different individuals. The public accounts therefore attend to the one factor that it is assumed individuals can control, which is their state of mind or their approach to life in general as well as to matters of health and illness, and in doing so they establish the moral criteria according to which individuals can be judged 'good' or 'bad' by others. The blueprint for the criteria which operate with respect to health and illness is derived from the attitude that people are expected to show towards employment. Thus 'good' people are not only hard-working, they are also cheerful and stoical and, if they feel ill, they prefer to work off their symptoms rather than give in to them. 'Bad' people, on the other hand, are people who will not work (malingerers) and who are also likely to be hypochondriacs who waste valuable medical resources.

The process of medicalization cuts across the discourse of commonsense in public accounts and weakens the force of the traditional (in Habermas's meaning of the term) stress on strength of character and moral fibre in relation to health. It has the effect of neutralizing the force of the moral arguments. If there is medical proof that the illness is either 'normal' or 'real', then the burden of responsibility for that illness – though not for the patient's reaction to the illness – is lifted from the patient. If there is no such proof, then the moral status of the illness remains problematic and has to be negotiated much more carefully.

Private accounts of illness

In the context of this discussion, the significance of the content of private accounts of illness is that they focus attention on the material concerns and practical constraints that intrude into matters of health and illness. Private accounts draw attention to the 'ground' on which medical ideas fall and in doing so indicate the significance of 'the state of readiness of individuals and sub-cultures' referred to earlier, which determines the rate of progress of the medicalization process.

The private accounts with which we are concerned here are of illness. There are no private accounts of health in the interviews. People did not spend time recalling periods of their lives in which they knew what it was to feel healthy, or talk about feeling well at all. When they were telling their individual medical histories, the moral concerns so much to the fore in public accounts faded into the background. They were there, but they were less prominent. The three categories of illness defined by their relationship to medicine, and by their potential for medical treatment, were relevant, but in private accounts they figured as only one element in a complex set of relationships and concerns which affected people's perceptions of symptoms and their responses to feeling unwell and other signs of illness. The exact configuration of factors determining any one person's experience of illness – meaning both their perceptions of symptoms and their response to them – varied according to their own particular circumstances, but three factors were regularly and consistently implicated. These were their employment position, their position in the sexual division of labour, and their past experience of health and welfare.

Almost invariably the private accounts of illness show that one or more of these three factors affect the way in which the person giving the account had felt or had dealt with their illness. It must be remembered, however, that idiosyncratic events and circumstances could also determine their experience of illness. To take one example: when she was in her twenties, Kathleen Read tolerated a series of startling and serious physical changes for a period of six months before contacting a doctor. Kathleen had worried about her symptoms. Her skin and hair had changed in texture and coarsened, her eyes had bulged and she had found herself unable to distinguish between forwards and back, up and down, and movements sideways. Her mother and her husband had both pressed her to consult a doctor but she had not done so because she was living away from London at the time, and she had plans to move which had not yet materialized. As far as she was concerned, once she saw a doctor she would become a patient, she would *be* ill, and she had not wanted this to happen until she was back in London where her children could be looked after by her mother and her married sisters. As soon as she did move back to Bethnal Green, Kathleen contacted a doctor and after lengthy out-patient investigations her condition was diagnosed as a deficiency of the thyroid gland.

The following examples of private accounts all involve men, and have been chosen because they illustrate the way in which their position at work affects how they think about their health and make decisions that affect it.

Daniel Mayes and Stan Flowers had both been woodworkers. Working with wood is potentially dangerous on three counts: damage to the limbs and the back can result from lifting heavy timber and machinery; accidents can result from the use of sharp blades in cutting machines; and the wood dust from cutting, planing, and sanding can cause bronchial damage and is known to be a carcinogen. Daniel had been employed in an establishment that was a trade union closed shop and was large enough to be visited by the Health and Safety Inspectorate. The firm kept to the safety regulations in the industry: dust extractors had been installed in the 'fifties, the machines had guards, and the men were provided with protective clothing and with milk, which is considered protective against the fine dust produced by sanding machines. Daniel had been in a senior position on the shop floor and had been able to pick and choose his jobs, and he had simply refused to work on the sanding machines because he considered them too dangerous. In his opinion the men who worked them were taking a risk, but it was up to them: 'you'll always find someone who'll do anything for money', was how he saw it. In the course of his time in that job he had one serious accident with a cutting machine which laid him off work for six months and has left him slightly disabled in one hand. In his view the accident had been his fault because he had not used the guard on the machine, and he had accepted that he would not get compensation. The reason he had not used the guard was that he had to do a fine piece of work in a hurry, and the use of the guard made it more difficult.

Stan Flowers worked in a workshop that was too small to accommodate extractors and where the men were not provided with protective clothing or with milk. Stan said he had two worries about the effect of his work on his health. One was that by using the heavy machinery he was damaging his back; the other was that he often felt congested after about an hour in the workshop. He also felt that he had no choice but to continue doing the same job:

'I used to get quite a bit of back-ache. That's due to the heavy machine, pushing it. Cross-cutter. I thought I'd have to go to the doctor's once over that. He told me, "Well, the only way to get rid of that is to pack up what you're doing". I said, "I can't do that".'

As Stan saw it, there was not the space to install extractors in the workshop as well as the machinery, and without the machinery he would not have a job to go to. He called the detrimental effects on his health 'occupational hazards', by which he meant hazards that were an inevitable part of the job: 'Well, it's something you get used to, I suppose. It's like a coal miner, isn't it? You accept it as a job, you call it a liability. It's the only job I know, anyway.'

When William Cox was interviewed, he was spending the major part of his working days and nights driving lorries, and he was worried about the effect this was having on his hearing and on his vision:

'It's sending me deaf. The noise of the engine. I come home and I can't hear the telly. If I've been out, not so much now because I am in the warehouse, but if I've been out all day driving, not a long way – say to Oxford and back which is like two, three hours out and two, three hours back – I come home and I can't hear the telly. I can hear it, but not as loud as I can. That's about the only thing it's doing to me, but, there again, it's the lorry. If it was a new lorry with a suppressed cab, you wouldn't be hearing the noise. It wouldn't be doing it.'
JC: 'Does it worry you?'
WC: 'It does a bit, yes. That part of it does. I don't really want to wear glasses, I don't know why, most drivers have to wear glasses. Whether it's the strain on the eyes or something. The guy next door, he's an ex-driver, and he's right deaf.'

As a child, William had suffered from eczema. This had developed into dermatitis and was aggravated by contact with the oil and muck of mending engines and machines. Although he knew he was deafening himself driving lorries with poor suspension, he also knew that the firm could not afford newer lorries and that without the lorries they had, they would be out of business:

'The lorry that I drive is a good lorry. It's roadworthy, the tyres are good, the brakes are good, the appearance of the lorry is good. But it's an L registration lorry which is eight years old, which is old for a lorry. The life of a lorry is about two, three years. The suspension in the cab has gone so like it's rough, it's not a comfortable ride in the lorry and there's play in the steering wheel which you have to – but everything on it is, it passes the MOT test. It's hard work driving the lorry. You get a brand new lorry up the side of it, it's comfortable, it's just like sitting in an armchair driving. But the company at the moment can't stand buying new lorries while we can buy them sort of lorries and I can do them up on Saturdays and Sundays and keep them on the road and still earn money that new lorries earn.'

His attitude towards his dermatitis was equally pragmatic. He was aware that there were preventive measures he could take to protect his skin when he was working, but they would slow him down and his priority was to do the work quickly:

'Over the Christmas holidays all that clears up because I'm not touching grease and oil. I could wear gloves at work all day and it would clear up, but there are certain things you can't do in gloves and, being like me own Guv'nor, if a motor breaks down in the yard or out on the road and I've got a set mind of a load that's got to go somewhere, it's down to me to do it. So I'm always the first one to get under the lorry when there's something to be done, so I don't normally worry about gloves. I always think I'll go and get another jar of cream or something.'

Finally, there was Mick Chalmers. In the past, he had worked with dangerous materials (asbestos) and in dangerous conditions, and in his present job as a drayman he was aware of the constant strain in handling heavy weights. Intermittently the job exposed him to more acute physical dangers:

'The top of me arm is killing me when I've finished because it's been hitting me so hard [the crates] – bash, bash and jolting. The arms ache after, especially if you catch two hundred cases off the end of the board. You get out and go, "sod that". When it rains, it's murder. Especially when you're putting the kegs down. You've got a twenty-two gallon keg. You put your hook on it, you put it over the hole and you hold onto the rope and lower it down. But the rope's soaking wet, the sticks are soaking wet. So as you put it over, the weight of it tears it down and you're hanging on to it. It just whizzes straight through your hands. And you've got to hang on to it because if it hits the bottom it bounces and it'd kill one of the blokes down the hole. Because some of these cellars are so small the bloke's only about three foot away from the thing when it hits the floor. If you don't hang on to it, if you just let it go, it hits and it shoots and it could kill him.'

One man had lost a finger and another had his toes broken in accidents like these since Mick had been working as a drayman. At any one time, 10 percent of the draymen were normally off sick with back trouble, dislocations, muscle strain, and other injuries. Mick himself had been off work twice in each of the past two years, and in the twelve months previous to the interviews he had been laid off twice, once for three weeks and once for ten weeks. The draymen had been shown how to lift and carry heavy weights without causing themselves injury but, according to Mick, they were unable to put these methods into practice when they were working. In the places where they did the lifting – on lorries and in cellars – there was not always enough physical space to move without twisting to get around corners, and if they followed the recommendation to lift heavy weights in pairs, the time allowed for the delivery rounds by the brewery would have to be increased. He was concerned about the possible long-term effects on his health of staying in the job, but preferred working to the only alternative he could see which was to be unemployed:

'I find I haven't got a lot of choice really. To tell you the truth, I'm thirty-nine now, I can't visualise myself being able to do this job when I'm sixty. So I can't actually look at it and say, "I could last out till I'm sixty-five here, and retire from here". The chances are I won't anyway because of the redundancies and all that, but when I look at it in the cold light of day, it might not be a bad thing being made redundant before I get much older. And then I'll have to find something else, won't I? Or if anything else crops up, or if it don't crop up. 'Cause I don't think I'll be able to last. I don't feel all that great now at thirty-nine, but I can imagine in twenty years' time how I'm going to react to this job. I'd hate to think the job is doing me back in so that in the end I'm going to suffer. I can put me hand to roughly anything if I have to. But there isn't actually a lot of work about where I could say to myself, "Okay, I'll jack this in and go and do that". Perhaps in five years' time the climate might be better and there might be plenty of jobs going about, a bit of choice what to do. At the moment I look at it that I haven't got much choice, I've got to do it.'

All the men showed a deep ambivalence in their talk of the hazards associated with their jobs. They accepted the risks as part of the job and had a certain amount of pride in having the strength and stamina to cope with them, pride that was caught up with images of masculinity and of being tough. They were also aware of the long-term implications of remaining in damaging environments but the extent to which they could envisage alternatives for themselves depended on their position in relation to employment generally. The only solution Mick Chalmers could see was redundancy, and he was partly ready to welcome it, but William Cox could envisage moving away from working directly with the lorries in the future, and moving into the financial and administrative sides of the business. For the present, what mattered to all of them was that the work was available and was there to be got on with.

The sexual division of labour which operates both inside and outside the home is another factor that determines the nature of people's experience of illness. The men and women involved in the study had very different responses to feeling unwell which were largely structured by their position in the sexual division of labour. The demands of employment are usually more contained, and more containable, than the demands of housework and child-care. For the men, therefore, the important question was whether or not they felt able to continue to go to work, and as long as they were able to, they did what they called 'working it off'. At home, however, they had no qualms about expecting their wives to be sympathetic whilst they 'gave in' to even fairly mild symptoms. They also seemed to have very little trouble in taking to their beds when they were at home so as to be fit for another day of 'working it off' at work. They expected the women to look after them because they were supposed to be responsible for health in the family, and as an extension of their normal domestic obligations. However, this was one responsibility that the women appeared to shoulder extremely reluctantly, certainly far more reluctantly than their responsibilities for the children's physical well-being. In fact, it was when they were complaining about how their husbands – 'it' as some women called them – behaved when they were ill, that the women came closest to making explicit their resentment of their endless domestic duties and of their husbands' behaviour generally:

> 'He sits there and what irritates me more than anything, I can be walking around with my head falling off my shoulders but I've still got to carry on. I've still got to see to the kids. And when I actually sit down, he sits there and he goes, "Oh, I've got a headache". And I say, "Yes, so've I". He goes, "Make us a cup of tea", and I say, "Well, I've just sat down. Can't you make one?" "Oh, I can't make one now, it's too much." I say, "If I laid down and died every time my head hurt me there wouldn't be much done".'

> 'Men, they're like babies. You don't know what I put up with from him. Women, they get on with it. I mean, I keep saying I have to work it off. There I am with a bad knee. Sometimes I can't get up those stairs and it's banging on the floor. "Cup of tea!", and I'm going, "Wear the old 'uns out first". Absolutely babyish and I think that would go for 99 percent of men. Most men are babyish, aren't they? They couldn't stand the pain. Especially labour pain, they'd never survive. They really wouldn't. They really are babyish. I'd say that women have more aches and pains than men, but, as I say, when you've got a family, you'll find a woman will work till she's dropping. But she'll do what she's got to do and then she'll say, "Right, I'm off to bed". Whereas it's all right for a man. If he's ill he's got nothing to do, he just lays there, doesn't he? And expects to be waited on hand and foot. I find if I'm ill, I could go out there and die and they wouldn't even know I was here. His idea is, "I'm in the pub out of the way". Even when the children were young, he'd take them out and be out all day and I'd have to get up and make a drink.'

Their own response to feeling unwell was very different, as the comments about 'carrying on' and 'doing what they've got to do' in these two passages indicate. Instead of trying to 'work off' their symptoms as the men did, the women tried to accommodate their symptoms in order to keep going. If they could not succeed in containing their symptoms and were quite unable to 'carry on', then they readily consulted a doctor in the hope of getting something that would put them back on their feet looking after the children. Because they were in command of their daily routines, if they felt unwell they would cut out certain activities and slow down, anything in order not to have to give up altogether, which would mean that there would be no-one to look after the children and no-one, as Peggy Freeman pointed out, to look after the women either. Mary Webb told a story about the period that preceded her admission to hospital for emergency treatment which was instructive for a number of reasons.

Mary's difficulties had started after she had been fitted with an interuterine device that had caused her to have fortnightly periods that lasted two weeks. She worried about the amount of blood she was losing but had not gone back to the Family Planning clinic where the coil had been fitted because it meant making an appointment, because the wait in the clinic was always long and the bus journey was complicated, and especially because she would have had to take the youngest children with her. After some months she began to feel very tired and weak and then developed a cough:

'I used to be like an old-age pensioner walking along and all of a sudden everything used to go round. I was walking along and everything used to go black and all lights used to come before my eyes.'
JC: 'How long had that been going on for?'
MW: 'A few months. Ever since this terrible cough I had, it was all connected with the lump in the throat, but it was lack of blood getting to the main arteries, well to the arteries, I should imagine, that was causing it all. [She had been later diagnosed as having a severe form of anaemia.] I think it's not laziness really, it's just that you think, "Oh, it could be worse than it is" so you try to push it to the back of your mind and just carry on.'
JC: 'Did Charlie know you were ill like that?'
MW: 'Yes, and he said, "Oh, your mother won't go to the doctor's or to the hospital no matter how much you keep on after her, she just won't go. But she should do. Wait until she's ill and then, you know, it's too late then." But when I went to the Hackney Hospital and they got the results of the X-ray and the blood test, as I say, they didn't even mention the lump in my throat, they were more concerned with this anaemia and they said, "We'll keep you in now".'

Mary had cut down on her housework and was only managing at all by moving extremely slowly, but she had not been sure whether she was suffering from a 'health problem that was not an illness', and her tiredness was simply the product of having too much to do, too many children to look after and not enough sleep, or whether she was 'really' ill. When she did contact her doctor it was because she had developed the small lump in her throat mentioned above. To her, the lump meant one of two things – cancer, or a malfunctioning saliva gland such as her sister had recently had operated on. The story is interesting because it shows how easily people can rationalize and accommodate themselves to symptoms if that is what they want to do, and also the importance of the definition of the illness as 'real' or 'not real' in the decision about what to do. Mary had not wanted to bother a doctor for something that was perhaps a sign of weakness or of lack of stamina on her part, but as soon as a 'real' symptom appeared, she had not hesitated.

Jackie Cox told a story in her interview that indicated a surprising readiness to consult a doctor, but again, for pragmatic reasons. Jackie's problem had been depression. It had started after she miscarried a pregnancy that she had very much wanted, and had lasted six months. After a while, Jackie had felt that it was going on too long and that she was being *unfair* to her husband and to her daughter for allowing it to continue. She consulted a doctor and asked for anti-depressants to get her over the last bit more quickly and to speed up the process of recovery. Jackie said at another point in her interview that she disapproved of women who take anti-depressants and tranquillisers all the time, and that she felt that this was a sign of weakness on their part. Depression, in her view, is not an illness, it is a health problem and the person who has it has to help themselves out of it. However, as she put it, her first priority had to be her responsibility towards other people (in this case her husband and one child), and this made her own visit to the doctor legitimate.

Finally, we come to the third factor – past experience of doctors and health services – which played a part in the private accounts of illness in the interviews. The organization of health services and the standards of treatment available to Tower Hamlets residents are outlined in Chapter 7. For the moment, we direct attention to the significance of age differences in private accounts of illness as an indication of generational differences in people's experience of the health service and of welfare in general.

The older people in the study – the Neagles, Nellie Davies, Ben Knight – attached more significance to moral calibre when they were talking about the nature of health, than the younger people who tended to attach more importance to external factors in health and illness such as germs and viruses and social stress (see Chapter 6 for a detailed discussion of aetiological theories in the interviews). Related to this, the older people were more reluctant than the younger people to use the health service at all, and the interviews contain many accounts of them, and of the older generation in every family, refusing to consult doctors when they were ill. In some cases this was related directly to something that had happened. Nellie Davies, for example, had asked for a home visit from her GP and had been visited by a doctor from the emergency service contracted to his surgery. The next time she had an appointment, her GP had reprimanded her for using the service unnecessarily, confirming her and her husband's belief that doctors 'don't care about old people'.

Generational differences have been observed in other studies (Blaxter and Paterson 1982; Helman 1978), where it has been suggested that the emphasis older people place on internal factors and their attitude of 'independence' towards doctors and towards medicine comes from having grown up outside the National Health Service. There may be other, more general differences in the social experience of the generations which are also significant. It is certainly true that Nellie Davies was afraid of doctors and particularly of hospitals, and that she insisted that if she was to go into hospital she would never come out again. However, conversations with the Neagles, and the reports of Arthur Davies and other men of his generation in the study families (e.g. Mick Chalmers's and William Cox's grandfathers) suggested another explanation. The kind of 'individualistic' ideology which encourages independence and exaggerates the moral significance of 'having the right attitude' towards life, is especially pertinent in situations in which people are faced with poverty and with other material hardships which they can do nothing about. 'Having the right attitude' – which, in this context meant being cheerful and hard-working, having stamina and being resistant — might therefore mean far more to the older people in this study who lived in slums and knew financial hardship which was not alleviated by a comprehensive system of state benefits.

It is not only the National Health Service, but the welfare state more generally that has made the difference. The lesson the older generation learned from their parents was self-reliance. They believe that it is up to them alone to take care of themselves and of their families, and they resent that aspect of the welfare state that they see sapping people's spirit of independence, encouraging dependence, and discouraging them from standing on their own two feet. To some extent, they have succeeded in handing these attitudes on to their children, but the younger people have grown up in a different physical and social environment and have not had the same experience. For the generation that grew up after the war, the National Health Service, council housing, and a state system of financial benefits are facts of life which they take for granted. Often the younger people share their parents' hostility towards particular branches of the welfare state (and particularly towards social workers – see Chapter 7), but the roots of their resentment are different. The older people object to the services themselves, whereas the younger people are critical of the way they are managed. The older people want as little to do with the services as possible, whereas the younger people want to get what they want out of them.

Conclusion

This chapter has introduced the concept of medicalization into the discussion and used it to interpret some of the material relating to matters of health and illness in the interviews. It has shown that in the interviews the meaning of concepts of health and illness varied according to the type of account the person was giving. In public accounts people were principally concerned with moral aspects of health and illness and with proving that they stood in the right relationship to them. In contrast, in the stories they told about episodes of illness in their own or other people's medical histories (i.e., in private accounts) their preoccupations were more practical and more pragmatic. Both types of account included scientific (medical) and normative (commonsense) legitimations for health and illness, but the public accounts demonstrated a much greater awareness of and concern with the authority of doctors and the medical profession over the field of health and illness generally than was evident in private accounts. One of the major differences between the two types of account in fact concerns the marked care people took in public accounts of health and illness not to stray too far from concepts and theories that they believed were medical or were compatible with medicine.

As yet, the comparative literature on lay concepts of health and illness in industrial societies is not very extensive (Herzlich 1973; Blaxter and Paterson 1982; Pill and Stott 1982; Williams 1983), but it does contain some common themes. This is not in itself surprising. To the extent that they are members of industrial societies, regardless of class background and country of origin, the subjects of these studies share a common, medicalized culture.

Their dominant conceptions of health and illness are medical. For example, one of the findings common to the various studies (the present study included), is the difficulty lay people have in defining what they mean by 'health' and 'being healthy'. It seems likely that this difficulty can be attributed directly to the fact that – unlike some oriental systems of medicine – Western medicine does not have a definition of health apart from health as the absence of disease.

Although some common themes have emerged from the studies that are available, the analysis put forward in this chapter suggests that it would be wise to be cautious about making generalizations about 'lay' or 'working-class' (most of the studies involve working-class subjects) concepts of health and illness, based upon them. There are two reasons for this. The first is that we do not know whether the common themes stem mainly from public or from private accounts, or from both public and private accounts. They often seem to originate in what appears to be public accounts, which makes it difficult to know whether they are to be interpreted as evidence of similarities in the way individuals from different social groups and sub-cultures respond to the authority of medicine and the medical profession, or as evidence that their commonsense ideas and theories about health and illness are in fact the same.

The second reason for caution is that we need to know the meaning of the other concepts with which health and illness are associated in the different social groups and sub-cultures that have been studied. It is not enough to know that health is interpreted as 'functional ability' or 'capacity to work' (see Blaxter and Paterson 1982; Pill and Stott 1982), without knowing something about the nature of the work people do and of their relation to it. For example: to an extent, the men and women who took part in this study share a common perspective on work and its moral significance, but to the men 'work' means their 'job' whilst to the women (most of whom also have jobs), 'work' means 'housework and childcare'. As a result, the conditions of what the men and the women take to be 'their work' are not the same and, as we have seen, the constraints operating on them when they feel unwell are also different. This example illustrates the importance of understanding the context in which concepts of health and illness are used in order fully to understand their meaning. If the contexts are not comparable, it is not likely that the meanings will be exactly the same, however much they may seem to be similar.

6 *The Causes of Illness*

Introduction

The previous chapter introduced the concept of medicalization and used it to analyse commonsense ideas about the nature of health and illness contained in the interviews. In this chapter the concept of medicalization is applied to the analysis of common-sense theories about the causes of illness (aetiological theories) put forward by people in the study. In this context, a theory is an intellectual concept which relates and makes sense of ideas about causal agents. The chapter reports both implicit and explicit aetiological theories. Much of the discussion is taken up with theories that were explicitly stated by the people who were interviewed, but attention is also paid to the conceptual frame-work underlying hypotheses about single aetiological agents.

Pill and Stott (1982) have brought lay aetiological theories to the forefront of recent medical sociological interest, with the argument that there is a connection between such theories and the success or otherwise of initiatives in health education, health promotion, and preventive health work. At present, and since the publication of *Prevention and Health: Everybody's Business* (Department of Health and Social Security 1976) the declared intent of state health policy in Britain is to emphasize and promote the principle of prevention rather than cure. The preferred strategy for achieving that aim is one that encourages individuals to take responsibility for their own health by giving up unhealthy activities and practices such as smoking cigarettes and drinking excessive amounts of alcohol, and adopting healthier ones such as taking exercise and following a sensible diet. Pill and Stott rightly point out that, leaving aside the question of whether or not the policy is desirable (see Crawford 1977 and Graham 1979 for criticisms of the policy for a 'victim-blaming' approach), its success will depend on how far the notion of individual responsibility for one's own health is acceptable to the general public. They write,

'The establishment of just what the concept of individual responsibility for health means to various groups in our society would seem to be a necessary first step in assessing how effective official policy on preventive health is likely to be and formulating appropriate strategies for behaviour change.' (Pill and Stott 1982: 43)

The question of what the notion of individual responsibility means to various groups is important in its own right but also as a specific case illustrating the general rule that health education/health promotion should address the concerns of the public it is trying to reach. Health educators and doctors must acknowledge that lay people have their own ideas and theories about health and illness and take account of them in the way that they approach the public. This argument is important; it is behind much of the current interest in lay aetiological theories in the social sciences (Pill and Stott 1982; Graham 1979; Blaxter and Paterson 1982) and has influenced the analysis of aetiological theories in the present study.

The theories about causes of illness which people put forward in their interviews differed according to whether they were part of public or private accounts of illness. In public accounts, aetiological theories were put forward in answer to direct questions about the causes of illness in general or particular instances affecting specific individuals. These were questions such as: 'When you think about the kinds of illnesses people whom you know well have had, do you see them as having been avoidable at any stage?'; 'Do you think these were illnesses they could have done something about?' and, with reference to an illness which had been mentioned in a medical history, 'What do you think caused that to happen?'. Public accounts were given when illness was the general subject on which discussion was focussed. In private accounts, aetiological theories were voiced either in the course of a person describing an episode of their own or someone else's medical history, or when the ostensible subject they were discussing was something other than illness, such as housing or a particular individual's personality.

The two types of account were distinctive for differences in their form and content that were consistent enough to justify defining them as 'public' and 'private' theories about the causes of illness. Public theories usually included a reference to 'they', meaning the medical profession, as in 'they say', or 'they know', or 'I've heard' or 'they don't know'; they were put forward assertively and with apparent conviction. In contrast, private theories appealed to no other authority than that of the person who was speaking or, occasionally, a relative with whom they had discussed the matter. They were suggested rather than asserted, often with a certain hesitancy. Public theories were addressed to the problem of who was to blame for the illness, which was never stated but was implicit in the way the theories were formulated. In most cases the problem was solved in such a way that the person who was ill was not blamed for the illness, and which allowed others to treat them with compassion. Very occasionally, public theories held persons responsible for their own illnesses, in which case other people were not expected to treat them sympathetically. Private theories explained the illness in terms of the person's life history but were much less concerned with the problem of responsibility for the illness and did not allocate blame.

The differences between the two types of account may be explained by the concept of medicalization as defined in Chapter 5 above. The distinctive characteristic of public theories is that they try to be, or to seem, medical in form and in content. The form and manner in which they were stated implicitly acknowledged medical authority in the area of health and illness. They were put forward with authority, but the authority the person claimed for their statements when they were theorizing publicly was medical authority (e.g., 'they say', 'I've heard', etc.), and not their own. The content of the public theories was thus an illustration of the interaction between commonsense (traditional) and scientific (modern) legitimations which characterizes the medicalization process. The overall framework within which the theories were couched was one that was concerned with the moral issue of responsibility for the illness, but this was solved – in the sense that the person who had the illness was absolved of the responsibility for causing it – by scientific concepts (or concepts that were thought to be scientific) being incorporated into the theory. This had the automatic effect of making the illness something 'other' from the person who had it, i.e., its cause was externalized. The illness was turned into an objective medical entity which existed apart from the person so that, in effect, it became a medical rather than a personal responsibility.

The causative factors in illness identified by public theories were always at one remove from the person; they were not things that people can know directly from their own experience. The most common explanations for illness in public theories involved concepts that were either borrowed directly from biomedical science (germs, viruses) or were close analogues of the causal factors identified in medical aetiological theories. For example, the notion of the individual constitution, which was often employed in public theories, is close to medical concepts of genetic susceptibility and congenital conditions; and the notions of stress, strain, pressure, and so on are close to the concepts of external stressors and stressful life-events contained in the growing literature on stress as a cause of disease. The result is that the conceptualization of the causal process in public theories had a static quality. Often it was a case of one thing causing the illness on its own, but if more than one causal agent was involved, the causal relationship was fixed in such a way that A acted on B (once) and produced the illness. This was further evidence of medicalization. The static quality in public theories partly resulted from the care people exercised in using ideas that were not necessarily their own, but it was also caused by the medical or quasi-medical character of the aetiological agents. When they were giving public explanations for illness, people were not reflecting for themselves on their personal experience, they were repeating theories they had heard and which they believed to be medically authorized. In contrast, the causative factors in private theories were events and incidents in people's lives and their personal relationships. The conceptualization of the causal process was dynamic rather than static, with many factors interacting – acting and reacting upon each other – and with illness as the eventual outcome.

These and other differences between public and private aetiological theories are explored at greater length in the rest of this chapter, which is divided into three sections. The first and second sections apply the concept of medicalization to a detailed analysis of the structure and meanings in public and private theories respectively, whilst the concluding section discusses the implications of this kind of analysis for health education/health promotion.

Public theories of the causes of illness

Medicalization – i.e., the interaction between commonsense and scientific legitimations in which the dominant part is usually taken by the latter – plays a part in the construction of public aetiological theories on a number of different levels. The background assumptions about the nature of illness on which the theories rest follow the tri-partite classification of illness into 'normal' illness, 'real' illness, and 'health problems that are not illness' which is legitimated scientifically. The previous chapter has shown that the classification takes some account of the severity of symptoms but is largely determined by the relationship of the condition to medicine and to how seriously it is taken by doctors.

The background assumption about the nature of health in public theories has *both* scientific and commonsense legitimation. The assumption is that inequalities in basic health are 'natural'; some people have better health than others because they are born with a 'better' or a 'stronger' constitution. The concept of the individual constitution is perfectly compatible with the medical theory of genetic susceptibility but it also fits with the common-sense theory that inequality is a natural phenomenon – whether it is inequality of intelligence and ability or inequality in health – which informs the attitude people in the study have towards employment and which they use to legitimate hierarchies of all kinds.

The interaction of commonsense and science in the content of the theories themselves is more complex. The theories are concerned with three different aspects of causation: the location of the causal agent (*place*); whether or not the condition could have been avoided (*circumstance*); and whether or not the person who has the illness is responsible for having it (*blame*). The three aspects are conceptualized as pairs of opposites: the agent can be *internal* or *external* to the person; the circumstances can be *avoidable* or *unavoidable*; and the person can be *blamed* or *not blamed* for having it. Logically, these six categories could be combined in eight different ways, e.g:

> internal/unavoidable/blame
> internal/unavoidable/no blame
> internal/avoidable/blame (and so on)

but in the public theories that were actually put forward in the interviews, only four combinations of categories were used:

1. internal/avoidable/blame
2. external/avoidable/blame
3. internal/unavoidable/no blame
4. external/unavoidable/no blame

The structure of the theories which people used was over-determined by the commonsense consideration of allocating blame for the illness, and the combinations of categories were in effect tautologous, i.e., different ways of saying the same thing. In the first two combinations the person was blamed because the illness was considered avoidable, in the second two the person was not blamed because the condition was considered unavoidable.

However, only the content of the first combination of categories was couched in uniquely commonsense (moral) terms; in the remaining three combinations the conceptual content of the categories was, or was intended to be, scientific. In the second combination (external/avoidable/blame) the person was held responsible for *having* the illness rather than *causing* it, and the element of blame was considerably diminished, whilst in the third and fourth combinations it was absent altogether. The significance of these points will become clearer as the analysis of the different combinations and their uses progresses.

The first combination of categories, i.e., internal/avoidable/blame was rarely used in the interviews. It explained mental health problems such as anxiety and depression, which people defined as 'states of mind' ('health problems that are not illness'), and problems of physical health if the person had allowed them to deteriorate very seriously. In the case of the latter, the initial cause of the problem may have been something for which the person, strictly speaking, was not held responsible, but they acquired responsibility by having allowed the condition to become 'unnecessarily' troublesome or painful.

Ann Cullen reported that she had suffered from anxiety and depression on and off throughout her adult life, and blamed herself for this. She saw the cause of her trouble with 'her nerves' as something inside herself which it was up to her to do something about. When the trouble began, she had been referred to a psychiatrist and at various times since then she had consulted her GP who prescribed tranquillisers. She kept a stock of pills in the house and took them when she felt it was necessary. Essentially, she said, her depression could be avoided, provided she was firm with herself and developed the strength of mind and the determination to overcome her own anxieties. This was what the psychiatrist had told her, and it was consistent with what she herself felt:

'I came out of the hospital. I came out of the London, and I walked home and all the way home I was saying to myself, "I ain't going in a madhouse". And this is what done it, from then on I was determined I wasn't going to end up – that's all I kept saying to myself, "Well, I'm not going in a madhouse" . . . It was only the fact of him telling me that if I'd gone on the way I was I'd end up in a mental home, and I thought, "No way, I'm not going there for anyone. I ain't leaving my baby." And I think this is what got me out of it to be honest with you.'

'It affects everybody differently, nerves. And I think nerves can be a very long-term illness. Because until you're ready to get yourself out of it, no-one else can. And they can give you all the tablets in the world and that will help, but it won't cure it. That's something you've got to do for yourself.'

Ann's theory of depression as an internally caused and avoidable state was shared by her daughter, Jackie, who had also had periods of depression. The emphasis in Jackie's discussion of the problem lay with the importance of acting responsibly in a situation for which, ultimately, she was to blame. Like her mother, Jackie regarded short-term use of tranquillisers and antidepressants as the responsible course of action, but both women disapproved strongly of women using drugs over long periods of time and, as they saw it, becoming dependent on them:

'I've had librium when I lived in Stevenage, but mainly I had them because of depression. 'Cause I was, 'cause things got on top of me out there. I've had them a couple of times. Not librium, but a few tranquillisers since I've been here, mainly when I consider, when major things have happened to me which –they may not be major to anyone else. Like when I lost the baby. I got myself over it pretty well, but it was just that last few steps, I couldn't quite get back to what I consider normal. I couldn't quite get back to the way I wanted to feel and I should've felt, so I went to the doctor's and he gave me some.'

Nellie Davies's family also used the first combination of categories to explain Nellie's ill-health. In effect they saw her condition as the product of hypochrondria; they believed that it was caused by her attitude towards herself and that it was therefore something that could be avoided, for which therefore she was to blame:

'She's always been ill, but it's her own bloody fault, she can't be bothered to go to the doctor's. She hasn't even got to go to the doctor's, she's on the phone. She's only got to phone over for the doctor to come over to her, but she can't be bothered. She don't want to go to a hospital because she's frightened she'll never come out. Which is ridiculous, because you don't have to stay on, they can do whatever they want to do, they can take tests as an out-patient.'

Nellie's relatives acknowledged in their interviews that forty years earlier her skin condition had been caused by an external agent. According to Joan Young it had been the detergent in which she used to soak her feet, and Kathleen Read said it had been caused by dye from a pair of shoes which had infected a blister on her foot. At that time she had consulted a doctor and been treated in out-patients, and the treatment she had been prescribed had worked. What they blamed Nellie for in the present was having allowed the illness to recur, and once it had recurred, for doing nothing about it and allowing it to become much worse.

The distinctive feature of this combination of categories in comparison with the other combinations, was the reference to personal motivation in the discussions about causes. The combination constructs theories that are similar to, but not the same as, psychosomatic theories of illness insofar as the illness is attributed to the person without the person's attitude or state of mind itself being regarded as a legitimate health problem (and thus in need, or deserving, of medical attention). Far from needng help or treatment for the way they felt, the person was blamed or blamed herself for indulging in behaviour that was generally considered reprehensible and disgraceful.

The second combination of categories (external/avoidable/ blame) was used rarely and only in relation to relatively minor episodes of 'normal' illnesses such as 'flus, fevers, colds, respiratory infections, and children's infectious diseases. In this context the external agent was always a germ or a virus which could have been avoided if the person had taken the proper precautions. Allowing oneself to catch cold or to get wet were the usual unnecessary risks with one's health that people described. Jeannie Moss, for example, said that when she was younger she had travelled home from the seaside in a wet bathing suit, and this had caused her to catch a chill which had later developed into pneumonia. Catching pneumonia had therefore been her fault. Some of the younger mothers in the group complained that other parents ignored the conventional periods of incubation and isolation for children's infectious diseases, and they blamed these 'other parents' for their own children catching diseases at school. In this instance they were shifting responsibility for their children's illness onto *someone else*, but the combination of categories making up their theory about why their children were ill remained the same.

The third and fourth combinations of categories (internal/ unavoidable/no blame, and external/unavoidable/no blame) were used more often than either of the other two and were applied to a much wider range of illness conditions including both 'normal' and 'real' illnesses. In the third combination, the internal causal agent was the 'constitution' of the person who was ill. Individual constitutions could either be weak, in which case the person would suffer from generally poor health, or they could be specifically vulnerable either to particular diseases or at a particular site, e.g., the heart, stomach, kidneys, etc. Differences in the quality of individual constitutions were explained in both commonsense and scientific terms. The commonsense explanation was that it was a matter of a person's 'luck' or of their 'fate' or 'destiny', or – sometimes – of God's will. The scientific explanation was that it was a matter of genetic inheritance, it was something that 'ran' in the person's family. In either case, the first indication of what the person's constitution was like was thought to be their weight at birth. The birth weights of every child in all the families were recorded and remembered meticulously. It was generally assumed that the heavier the baby the stronger its constitution, although Kathleen Read reported that in her case, the theory had broken down. She had been 'massive' as a baby (a point her sister, Mary, confirmed: 'she was always the biggest one of us, like fatness and things like that. Not the tallest, but she was fat. Roly-poly she was when she was small.'). However, Kathleen's adult health had been extremely poor. Kathleen's own theory was that it had been her fate to have had a hard life; she called it 'luck':

'Right through life I was the one that went down with lung trouble, I'm the one that's had a gland out, I'm the one who's had me womb out. Me, I'm the hospital case . . . If it's anything that's going to happen, it's going to happen to me sort of thing. I lost me husband first, didn't I? I was only thirty-nine when he died . . . Think that I had to go to a special school and that I could go blind by twenty-one, but if I hadn't gone blind by twenty-one all right, they wouldn't improve. So I suppose I'm lucky there, really, aren't I? In a way.'

Obviously, the premature death of Kathleen's first husband had nothing to do with her own constitution, but she included it in a list that was otherwise made up of her own health problems because it was part of the same 'luck' which made her prone to ill-health. It was that predisposition towards illness that Kathleen's sister, Mary saw as the reason why some people got ill and not others:

'What will be will be. And these different illnesses happen to anybody. I mean to say, I'm here, I feel as right as rain, but I don't know how I'm going to be in nine months or a year's time. See? So I think life is life, and if you're unlucky enough to pick up one of these diseases, it's just one of those things in life. You won't be able to prevent it, so really and truly it's the way your life is . . . Some people pick up these illnesses so quickly. And you don't know what starts it all off and what causes it until you go and have all these different tests done. But anybody can pick up these different diseases, and when it happens you hear people saying, "Oh, I didn't think it could happen in my family".'

Betty Mayes and her sister, Ann, had a very similar notion of 'fate' or of 'destiny' which they used to explain 'real' illnesses:

BM: 'My brother-in-law who died [of cancer], no-one could have been looked after better. She used to give him honey every morning. They never had no children, he had the best of everything. Before that man went out to work, he used to have honey and all that. It didn't save him, did it? If your body's made that way, it doesn't matter what you do. Nothing can alter your body, can turn your body another way. That's what I always say. If you'll be ill and you're to die, I always say, no-one can save you.'

AC: 'To me, I look at it this way. My life was already plotted out for me when I was born. And what's going to happen to me will happen to me. Whether I smoke, whether I drink, whatever I am, that will happen to me. And that is the way I look at it. And I think illness as well. You were born and your life's already plotted out.'

The idea of life 'already being plotted out' and of that being 'how it was meant to be' was expressed in other ways in the interviews, usually in metaphors about the 'luck of the draw' and 'your number coming up' and your name 'being in His [i.e., God's] black book'. But people who used these turns of phrase also had a scientific understanding of the notion of the individual constitution, which they discussed as a matter of genetic inheritance. Betty Mayes, for examle, said that her mother had been a diabetic and therefore all her children had inherited a vulnerability to diabetes (three of her brothers and sisters were diagnosed diabetics). Eddie Cullen, Ann's husband, had a brother and a sister who each had a heart attack and he had a nephew who had died from heart disease. Ann believed that this meant that the whole family was susceptible to heart disease and she had asked her GP to have Jackie and Jackie's children tested in some way to find out if they were especially at risk so that if they were, they could do something about it, such as making changes in their diet. The GP had refused on the grounds that it was unnecessary and, when she was interviewed, Ann was consoling herself with the thought that children inherit more from their mother's side of the family than from their father's and that this would afford Jackie and her children some protection:

'I know they normally say, when you have a baby, if there's any diseases they go more on the mother's side than they do the father's, they reckon, 'cause it comes – like you have the baby. So when you're pregnant and you go to the hospital, they ask all the information about your side of the family, not so much the in-laws.'

The concept of each individual having his or her own particular and unique constitution was thus legitimated in both common-sense and scientific terms. If we compare the two quotations above from the interviews with Ann Cullen, we can see the process of 'switching between' traditional and scientific (aetiological) theories which Habermas identifies as the outcome of rationalization/medicalization. In the one she expresses a purely traditional point of view, whilst in the other she appeals to medicine to legitimate the scientific theory she is putting forward.

The meaning of the internal/unavoidable/no blame combination, which is important in the sense that it affects what happens to people when they are ill and what they do about it, is that the person who has the illness is not blamed for it. There is, therefore, nothing that is personally expected of them other than that they should seek 'proper', i.e., medical, attention. The combination was often used to explain the more serious conditions that were discussed. Kathleen Read's thyroid deficiency, Ben Knight's brain tumour, Sarah Chalmers's nephew's epilepsy, and all cancer, heart disease, and diabetes in the families of Betty Mayes and Ann Cullen, as well as in other families, were explained in this way.

In the fourth and final combination of categories employed in public aetiological theories (external/unavoidable/no blame), the causal agent was either biological or social. The biological causes of illness were germs and viruses and also toxins and pollutants of various kinds such as fumes, asbestos, and lead in the air. The social causes were variously conceptualized as shocks, pressures, stress, strains, and worries. This combination accounts for serious infectious disease and for the modern diseases, cancer and heart disease. Where the cause was biological, people often said that the illness 'just happened'. Joe Hutchinson's children all had infectious hepatitis, for instance, for no apparent reason. Even if it did not just happen and the reasons why it had happened were obvious, it remained nobody's fault. Joanne Goode's son had, as a baby, been treated in an isolation hospital for an infection of the skin and bowels which had first appeared to be nappy rash. This was at the time when Joanne's marriage was breaking up and she was living in accommodation without heating and with no indoor toilet or hot running water. She was short of money and was eating badly. According to Joanne, the circumstances meant that the child had become ill, but they also meant that there was nothing that she personally could do about it. Neither she nor anyone else was to blame. Jackie Cox had dysentery as a child which she said she had caught from living in Russia Lane before the tenements were pulled down. Again, since this was where the family had been living, this made the condition unavoidable; the important point in this instance, as in the previous one, being that no-one, not Joanne, and certainly not the baby, not Jackie or her parents, could be held *personally* responsible for the fact that the illness occurred.

Where the causal agent was social in origin, it was conceived at such a high level of generality that it was again considered unavoidable and no-one was to blame. The 'pace of modern life' was a metaphor for a variety of factors including the quality of the food that is available, financial insecurity, anxieties about work and about unemployment which people said contributed towards cancer and heart disease:

DM: 'I wonder if it – I wouldn't say fast living, but living at a faster pace than our fathers did, and our mothers. 'Cause it is speeded up a hell of a lot really. Because, as I say, with the dancing and the rock and roll and boogying. And with probably drinking and even foods. I mean, to me, now, what did you get out of a tin? Probably condensed milk, yes? But now everything comes either in a tin or a packet. You throw it in the fridge and forget it. Get it out. And probably, I don't know, I don't think there's the same nutriment in the food. The animal flesh you got was fresh. Like it went in the cold for a spell. Now you've got to have hens that are laying a thousand eggs a week and then they destroy them because they've earned their keep anyway, that's it.'

KR: 'It probably does put a strain on your heart where everything is such a rush. Let's face it. I mean, you've only got to walk into the street and everything is hustle and bustle around you. 'Cause years ago everything was just sort of a slow and trendy [sic] plod, wasn't it? Your horses and carts. All right, I'm going back a few years, but even people sort of – I mean their attitude was a lot slower. You walk around now, time's precious to everybody and they're all dashing about here, dashing about there. I suppose it's going to take a strain on your heart eventually.'

JG: 'The cancer is coming down younger and younger. It's the same with heart complaints. I don't think it's always because you're overweight and you're not getting a lot of exercise. It's the pressure of life that causes a lot of – you look at the one that's just had [a heart transplant operation], he's twenty-three years old and he's had two attacks and yet you look at him. He's not fat and overweight so you can't turn round and say it's that. All right, maybe he's got a heart defect. Maybe it's the pressures of life. You find a lot of men have ulcers in their thirties now, where at one time it was men in their fifties and sixties. It's the pressure of life which causes it more than anything else. And there's no way you can take the pressures away because everyone's got it, everyone worries about money.'

The most common explanations of cancer in public theories, however, involved a *combination* of an internal predisposition towards the disease and some kind of external 'trigger' or shock which precipitates onset of the disease. Many people expressed the view (attributed to medicine) that everyone has cancer and cancer patients are simply the unlucky ones in whom the disease is activated:

AC: 'I was always of the understanding that it was brought on more by shock, they reckon, than anything else. If you have a shock, a bad shock, they reckon it can bring it out in a body, because we've all these diseases in our bodies, but it's only a matter of being brought out.'

JG: 'I think with something like cancer they don't really know enough about it yet, it's still one of those things that there's a lot of research on. They still don't know what causes it. I mean, they turn round and say everyone's got cancer of a kind, it just takes something to aggravate it.'

MC: 'Well, I've been told that everyone has got cancer inside them. You've got cancer, everyone's got it. It just needs something, to start it off, like a shock or something.

PF: 'You hear so many different versions. I would be inclined to believe that a knock could start off this growth and – I don't think, all right, it could be a virus, but I think a knock could start off this growth. And then I imagine it being like something inside with tentacles spreading all around. That's how I imagine it. A knock could start it off, a knock could liven it up.'

One fairly widespread belief was that medical intervention can be the trigger which sets the cancer off:

MW: 'I think once they take these different tests, cutting a bit off here and a bit off there, and they open you up, I think they liven the cancer up. And from then on you don't stand a chance, really.'

MC: 'Well, I don't know a lot about it, but when someone says to me "cancer", it's a thing that grows inside you and just eats you away. 'Cause everyone that gets it, they all lose weight. You lose weight straight away, so it must be something that eats you away inside. And I think it just eats and eats and eats until you get so weak you can't fight it any longer and you die. 'Cause I've heard of people, some people they catch cancer and it seems to take a long while before they die. And yet I've heard of other people catching it and dying quick . . . But I know one thing. If I went to the doctor's and he said, "You've got cancer, come in and have it cut out", I know I wouldn't go in and have it cut out. 'Cause I know a few people that have been in, and they've had cancer and been cut and they've still died. Cutting it, I think is the worst thing to do. 'Cause just talking to people in general, it seems to make it more active when they start cutting it. They do seem to live longer if they don't have it cut about than they do if they've had it cut.'

There is a curious paradox about this belief in the harmfulness of medical treatment of cancer which was one of the few ways in which people in the study demonstrated that they had reservations about modern medicine and were frightened by it. In most other contexts, they showed an uncritical belief in the efficacy of medicine, but in this instance, medicine was identified with the 'modern way of life' which is in itself a threat to people's well-being (see Herzlich 1973: 37–8). The other way that people expressed the opinion that medicine might be dangerous was by talking about how they or other patients had been treated as 'guinea pigs'. Kathleen Read, for example, said that one of the hospitals that had treated her first husband's tuberculosis had been doing experimental operations on patients and that her husband had discharged himself from the hospital rather than be used as a 'guinea pig'.

Where the external causal agent in the aetiology of an illness was identified as a virus or a germ, the scientific legitimation is clear. The sources of legitimation for the social causes mentioned in public theories are more ambiguous, and it is perhaps significant that it was when they were theorizing the relationship between the internal constitution of the person and the shocks, pressures, triggers etc., which might 'bring on' the cancer that people most often claimed medical authority for their words. This was partly perhaps because they were discussing a 'real' illness and might have been thought to be 'trespassing' on medical territory, but it was also because the status of concepts of stress, pressure, worries, and so on is ambiguous. There are common-sense notions of stress and pressure which express people's experience and understanding of their relation to their external environment, but at the same time people are becoming aware that such concepts are increasingly being used in medical and epidemiological research into the causes of 'real' illnesses, i.e., cancers and heart disease.

However, the lesson of public theories that identify external agents, or combinations of internal agents and external triggers, in the aetiology of disease as far as people in the study are concerned, is that the person who has the disease cannot be blamed for having it: it is unavoidable. 'Shocks' are by their very nature idiosyncratic and therefore unpredictable, and it is assumed that stress and pressure is a fact of life – almost a 'natural' feature of life in modern urban and industrial environments. The implications of this position for health education and prevention are considered in the concluding section of the chapter. For the moment the significance of this final combination of categories in public aetiological theories is that, in general, the response to patients with serious 'normal' and 'real' illnesses is wholly compassionate. No-one thinks to say that the illness could in any way have been their fault because, by definition, it is something they could not have avoided. It is noteworthy also that social causes are conceptualized at such a high level of generality that nothing and no-one else is to blame.

Private theories of the causes of illness

Compared with the number of public theories, there are very few private theories of the causes of illness in the interviews. The material in this section is gathered together from parts of the interviews in which illness was not often the focus of discussion, because as soon as it became the focus, people tended to express themselves in public theories which sounded appropriately medical.

Private theories can best be described by telling the stories in which they appeared. One of their characteristic features, for example, was that the dichotomies between internal/external, avoidable/unavoidable, and blame/no blame, around which public theories were constructed, disappeared altogether. Instead of the cause being either internal or external to the person, or, as in the theories about cancer described above, internal *with the addition of* an external trigger, private theories hypothesized a *causal process* in which there was *movement between* factors internal to the person and factors external to them and in their environment. In this context the question of whether or not the illness was avoidable did not have the moral significance of public theories, because the illness was not portrayed as something that could be separated from the person or the circumstances of their personal biography.

The story Mary Webb told about her brother's illness illustrates

these points. The story began with Arthur (junior) being cons-
cripted into the Navy in the Second World War and catching
jaundice which damaged his liver. Arthur loved having a good
time – he had been the organizing force behind family parties –
and he was much liked at work and amongst his friends generally.
It was part of his personality to be sociable, and part of being
sociable was that he drank a lot. As a result of the quantities of
alcohol he consumed, Arthur developed an illness which was
eventually, according to Mary, diagnosed as cancer of the liver.
He was admitted to hospital for exploratory surgery and died
shortly afterwards. Mary said that ultimately she believed it was
the surgery that had killed him:

> 'I think it's opened up and I think it must start the disease really
> getting a grip and it just travels round your body so quickly.
> More than likely, Arthur, he might have died, but more than
> likely he would've had a few more years with us if he hadn't
> have had that first. It must start something off, I think, though
> he was in terrible pain, he had to have something done. He was
> in shocking pain all the time.'

The surgery was the last in the series of events that had caused
Arthur to be ill in the first place. None of them was his fault, but all
of them could have been avoided. The story specified the factors
involved in the illness sufficiently precisely for it to be possible to
ask, 'what if?'. What if Arthur had not been called up? What if he
had not been such a heavy drinker? What if he had not had
surgery? This feature of private theories, of being able to ask,
'what if?' *without implying blame*, is illustrated further in the
following story about Arthur Davies senior.

The public theory of Arthur Davies senior's amputated leg was
that he had developed gangrene because that was how his body
was made (it was simply the result of a constitutional defect) and
there was nothing anyone could have done about it. However,
Kathleen Read and her sister, Mary, suggested at various times in
their interviews that their father's illness had really been caused by
the circumstances surrounding the death of his eldest son and by
more recent events in his own life. The death of his son had come
as a great blow to Arthur senior. Some years earlier, he and Nellie
Davies had been moved from their rented terraced house into a
council flat on a busy road and without a garden. Neither of them
liked the flat and both of them missed the garden. They felt lost
without it and without other members of the family living with

them. The conflict and tension which had always been a feature of their relationship worsened, and Arthur withdrew himself to the pub whilst Nellie withdrew into her real and imagined illnesses.

Arthur's most regular drinking companion was his eldest son, and when he died, he lost the only relative he was close to. According to Kathleen he had reacted to his son's death by saying that it should have been him who had died, and he had felt guilty that he had gone on living. He refused to talk about his son with the rest of the family, and eventually was not talking to them about anything at all. Around the same time, Nellie's skin condition worsened and the episode reported in the previous chapter, in which she had been reprimanded by her GP for requesting a home visit, occurred. That episode confirmed Arthur's antipathy towards doctors generally, and it was then that he announced that 'doctors are not interested in old people'.

As a result of his isolation at home and his resentment of doctors, Arthur did not report the fact that he had pain in his toe and foot to anybody until three weeks after he first noticed it. When the pain was unbearable and he could no longer walk on it, he told the son-in-law who had become his most regular, if infrequent, drinking companion, and made an appointment to see the GP. Further delay ensued because the GP gave him a letter of referral to the local hospital and he was given an out-patient appointment for two weeks' time. He was eventually admitted as an emergency into the hospital before the two weeks were up; gangrene was diagnosed immediately and the leg was amputated well above the knee.

In this story, there are many points at which it is possible to ask 'what if?' without blaming Arthur for becoming ill. What if he had not been forcibly re-housed? What if his relationship with his wife had been different? What if he had been able to share his grief with someone in the family, or an outsider, and had not cut himself off from the rest of the family? What if the GP had not so offended him that he had vowed not to ask for medical help? What if there had not been the delay of a few more weeks, would he have lost his foot rather than the entire leg?

In these private theories about what caused particular illnesses to occur in particular people, the causal factors are recognisable events and situations in the personal biography of the patient. This is in contrast with public theories where the causal factors are things people 'know about' rather than know directly. It is one thing to know about a person's drinking habits or about what the death of their son meant to them or of how they reacted to being re-housed, and quite another to have ideas about the composition of their constitution, or about germs and viruses or the vague and intangible stresses and pressures of 'modern life'. The relationship between the individual and the environment in private aetiological theories is dynamic: the illness is seen as the product of a causal chain of action and reaction which takes place over time; in public theories the same relationship is static: the illness is the product of internal *or* external causes, or of the unidentifiable coming-together of the two at an unspecified moment in time. It is not the case that private theories stand outside the medicalization process altogether. Illness is classified in the same way: 'normal' illness, 'real' illness, and 'health problems not illness', and there is a definite awareness of medical authority in the area of health and illness, which was apparent in the tentative way with which people in the study put forward their own views. But the moral problem of allocating responsibility and blame for the illness is largely irrelevant, and there was no attempt on the part of the people being interviewed to claim medical or any other authority for what they were saying when they were putting forward private aetiological theories.

Aetiological theories and prevention

The implications of public and private aetiological theories for the way in which people in the study approach the question of whether or not illness can be prevented are very different. The implications of public theories were indicated in the answers people gave in their interviews to a question about the Health Education Council's 'Look After Yourself' campaign. The question was purposefully introduced into the interviews to investigate attitudes towards prevention. Most people had heard of the campaign and were familiar with the bouncing figure that had been used to promote it. If they did not know about it, it was explained to them that the campaign argues that 'looking after yourself', i.e., not smoking, not drinking excessive amounts of alcohol, eating properly, and taking exercise can help to prevent heart disease and some cancers.

Daniel Mayes and his son, Andy, were the only people in the study who agreed with the campaign. Everyone else disagreed with it, but from different points of view. The most frequent response to the question about the campaign was to say that there is nothing anyone can do to prevent themselves becoming ill because, as Mary Webb argued in the quotation above, 'what will be will be' and 'these things just happen'. For Kathleen Read, it was a question of the person being able to do very little about their basic constitutional make-up:

'Well, I suppose it all depends if there's anything wrong with you in the first place. If you're a healthy person and you've done them sort of things, probably you would keep healthier a lot longer, or more years. But there again, you never know, you might go and catch a complaint from a kid and then – you think if adults catch kids' complaints, which is quite feasible, it doesn't matter how healthy you are, you're still going to get them.'

Ann Cullen objected to 'looking after yourself' in the way the Health Education Council advocates on the grounds that it encourages a morbid attitude towards oneself and one's health which is in itself likely to make one ill:

'The way I look at it, if you're not going to die of cancer or anything else, you're still going to die of something. You can't be a health fanatic all your life, can you? Let's be fair. What life would you have? You'd have none, would you? Some of the shit the health foods say what you've got to eat, what you've not got to eat. How can you live on it? You wouldn't get no pleasure out of it . . . I think with a lot of these campaigns lately, with all that's going on, if you took notice of them, you wouldn't eat. Let's face it. The cry came out, butter caused a bad heart. This caused a bad heart, that causes cancer, this causes cancer. If you listened to all of those, what would you do? What would your life be? You can't go through life saying to yourself, "I mustn't eat that. And I mustn't do this, and I mustn't do that." Because you've got no life, have you?'

Ben Knight argued in similar vein that 'health education' was a contradiction in terms if it meant that someone else could claim to know more about a person's health than the person concerned:

'If you want to give your life away and give people – tell them tell you what to do, you might as well tell them how to shoot yourself. You'd just as well be – why don't these people shoot themselves? Mentally unbalanced you say? Is it worry? Do you worry because you smoke too much? And people tell you you're going to die of cancer? Do you worry because they turn round and say, "You mustn't do this, you shouldn't do that?" If you did, where would you fetch up? . . . No-one can tell you how to rule your life or your destiny. I couldn't tell my children. I've learnt them the best way I can, but if they've got to learn, they've got to learn the same way I did. If they think smoking's harmful, or if they think drinking's harmful, or if they think they shouldn't eat too much. It always amazes me, it amazes me when people tell you, "you shouldn't do this". The only people that earn money out of life are people that tell you what to do and what not to do.'

Ben's idea that self-reliance and independence of mind were the first principles of good health was echoed by Jackie Cox:

'It doesn't matter what you do, you could go out and jog every day and have a heart attack for no reason. You know? I mean, you've got to live life the way you want to and the way you feel you can push yourself. I mean, if you smoke, say like you smoke and drink, if you drink and you know that you've got something like, you know, it'll make your blood pressure go up and make you ill, then when you get to the point, surely your own conscience will say to you, "Now stop it. Now. You're going to be ill otherwise." Obviously. Surely you mustn't go on until you're ill. No, I can't see the point of it, not really.'

Other people disagreed with the content of the Health Education Council's argument. Twenty-two people out of the twenty-four in the study said that they did not believe that smoking causes lung cancer. Twenty of them smoke twenty or more cigarettes a day. Most of them said that smoking might aggravate a pre-existing cancer, but based their disagreement on the argument that they know poeple who smoke and have not died prematurely, and have known people who did die prematurely but did not smoke. Harry Read died of cancer of the lung, but Kathleen refused to believe that cigarette smoking could have caused it, partly because in the early days (i.e., the nineteen-twenties and thirties) cigarettes had been sold on the wards of the Chest Hospital, but mostly because she had always smoked a great deal more than him:

'Well, if you was thinking about cancer, I'm going to turn round and say, "No". Because they said at the Chest Hospital when I lost Harry, they turned round and said he was a smoker. I said, "Well, if you're going to blame smoking, I would be the one with cancer and not him". Because what he smoked was very little. He used to have an ounce of tobacco and it'd last him about ten to twelve days, which is not heavy smoking.'

Mick Chalmers said his father had smoked all his life and is now, at the age of seventy, permanently out of breath. Mick's argument, however, was that 'they' might as well say, 'smoke thirty cigarettes a day and live till you're seventy' as say that smoking causes lung cancer and premature death.

Standard interpretations of these and other public responses in the interviews to the concept of illness being preventable by taking the appropriate precautions might be that people were *rationalizing* their resistance to changing their lifestyle, or that they were *fatalistic*. Neither observation is particularly helpful, however, if one is attempting either to understand why they reject the Health Education Council's message or to plan more effective educational strategies (see Salzberger 1976). In some cases people clearly were resistant towards changes in their drinking and smoking habits, but they were explicit about their reasons for not changing. William Cox, for example, had been persuaded that alcohol assists certain disease processes and thought that he ought to drink less. However, he continued to stop at the pub and drink three or four pints on his way home every night because, he said, it helped him to relax and this meant that when he came in from work he was much more able to cope with his family than he would have been otherwise. Kathleen Read was one of the heaviest smokers in the group and one of the many who said she would like to give up smoking for financial reasons and because she felt it made her chest tight. She had tried and had succeeded in cutting down on the number of cigarettes she smoked, but in stressful situations she *preferred* to smoke rather than feel tense:

'I smoked more when I was carrying Sally, and yet she was the biggest out of the four. She was seven pounds fourteen born, my Joanne was only five eleven. I was smoking like a trooper when I had Sally. In fact, I was doing about sixty a day, I think. To me and to my girls it was laughable. They turned round and said, "The way you're smoking, Mother, you'll have a yellow baby". You know? Because I was, literally, one after the other. And yet she turned out the biggest of them and nothing wrong with her.'

JC: 'Why were you smoking so much then?'

'Nerves probably. Well, as I turned round and said, I never wanted her anyway at that time of my life. And probably wondering how I was going to cope more than anything else, probably, and then knowing you've got to have the womb out, which usually takes about a year to get over. You think, well you've got a baby, how are you going to be able to cope? And everything used to build up so I really used to puff away. As I say, she was quite healthy. Seven fourteen, it's not exactly a small baby, is it?'

These were *explicit rationalizations* which explained why the person concerned did not change what they were doing even though they felt they ought to. They were quite different from the *empirical objections* to the theory that smoking causes cancer which amounted to a refusal to accept that the medical point of view is necessarily right.

Was it because people in the study did not understand the statistical reasoning behind the medical argument? Certainly this was Daniel Mayes's explanation for the difference between himself and his son, Andy (who accepted the medical argument), and his wife Betty who refused to believe that smoking was bad for her and continued to smoke forty cigarettes a day when Daniel himself had given up. However, it is not a convincing explanation because some medical theories have been accepted and become part of commonsense theorizing about the causes of illness without being fully understood. The commonsense version of germ theory, for example, is simpler and more literal than the scientific version and ignores the complicating factor that not everyone who is exposed to the same germ necessarily becomes ill. In contrast, the commonsense response to the medical argument connecting lifestyles and diseases was to *reject* it out of hand, and it is this that made it different. Thus the real question is why only some medical theories are accepted and become part of commonsense?

The notion of fatalism does not supply the answers. The meanings associated with fatalism in the social sciences include a belief in fate; an inability to project forward into the future which produces a 'present orientation'; an inability to take action on one's own behalf; and passivity and resigned acceptance of one's lot in life. Many people in this study were fatalistic in the sense that they believed in fate and accepted their lot in life, but far from reducing them to passivity that belief meant that they placed great importance on being active and making the most of it and getting the best out of life. This applied to their attitudes towards health and illness as much as to other aspects of their lives. Kathleen Read, for example, had a longer and more complex medical history than anyone else in the study which she attributed to her fate and her own bad luck, but she was far from being passive in general or in relation to her health. If she believed that there was something that could be done to improve her health she did it, but if she believed that there was nothing to be done then she actively set about adapting herself in whatever way necessary. For example, she had been told by her GP that there was nothing that could be done to help her rheumatism and arthritis and she had therefore decided to do what she could to alleviate the pain by soaking her joints in warm water and taking pain-killers, and to set herself to learn to put up with it. On another occasion, however, she had been told by her gynaecologist that she could expect to be incapacitated for up to a year after having a hysterectomy, and she had been appalled to witness a neighbour take almost this long to recover from the same operation. Kathleen's daughter was three months old when she had the operation and she had no option but to look after her when she came out of hospital. She prided herself on her recovery which took less than three months. It is not helpful to describe the people in the study as fatalistic simply because many of them said that they believe in fate, if it means overlooking the premium they themselves attach to taking the initiative in relation to health problems which is part of their approach to life as a whole.

The context in which their resistance to the 'Look After Yourself' campaign is best understood is that of medicalization. Until fairly recently, the trend of medicine and of what was understood of medicine was one that made illness into disease and thereby into something that was separate from the person who was ill. The causes of illness were increasingly identified as things known only to science — germs and viruses, toxins and poisons, genes and congenital conditions, and even the vague terminology of distress reactions and stress-related disease – and things that were therefore not the responsibility of patients. The whole trend of the Health Education Council argument – and, to take it wider, of state health policy – has been to reverse the direction in which medicine seemed to be leading. It is this reversal that people in the study will not accept because by making individuals responsible for their diseases, it conflicts with their most fundamental attitudes and moral beliefs.

The framework within which illness is publicly discussed is one that is dominated by a commonsense concern with questions of responsibility for illness and of what ought to be done about it. The aetiological theories which have been incorporated into that framework from medicine are ones that excuse the person who is ill for having the illness and pose medical treatment/intervention as the solution to the problem. This is not true of all aetiological theories in public accounts of illness, but it is true of all aetiological theories that explain illnesses that people in the study take seriously. Theories that make the patient responsible for their illness, i.e., psychosomatic and behavioural theories which call for individual solutions to the problem, have largely not been accepted. The reason for this is that the basic elements that make up the framework of public aetiological theories come from, or originate in, other areas of people's experience. The similarity between their commonsense ideas and theories about work and employment and their theories about health and illness, and the close connection between work and health explored in previous chapters, suggests that attitudes towards health and illness are principally formed by experience of employment and how that is interpreted. Certainly, the basic elements are the same: the acceptance of an unequal, hierarchical, and largely immutable 'natural order of things' and the emphasis on right-mindedness, cheerfulness, and positive thinking as the one contribution the individual can make towards improving his or her own lot in life.

Unlike public aetiological theories, the private aetiological theories of illness reported above offer several possible points of intervention for health education/health promotion. For example, in the case of Arthur Davies senior, the following events and incidents in his life were mentioned as factors contributing to the onset of disease: forced rehousing in a maisonette flat which was on a busy road and had no garden; the breakdown of communication between Arthur and the rest of the family following the death of Arthur's son and Arthur's inability to express his grief; the behaviour of the local GP. These factors are specific and, without implying blame, they do not appear to have been inevitable. This is important because it means that in contrast with public theories in which the aetiological agents *either* appear inevitable *or* imply individual responsibility for the illness, the conceptual space is generated in which it is possible to imagine arresting or reversing the disease process. The private theories thus provide possible starting points for health educators/promotors to begin to make the links which need to be made between individuals' state of health and their material and social circumstances.

7 Doctors and Health Services

Introduction

This chapter describes the attitudes that underlie the relationships that people involved in the study have with doctors and health services. The chapter does not attempt to provide an accurate record of their use of services, but it does refer to their experiences as patients. Attitudes towards health services, at least in part, are formed in response to the experiences people have as patients (Blaxter and Paterson 1982: 156). The process of feeling one way or another about a doctor, a clinic or a hospital, consulting the doctor, attending the clinic, and having that feeling either altered or confirmed, is interactive and it is not possible fully to understand attitudes without referring to the experiences with which they are connected.

The research methods employed in this study were not suitable for investigating people's actual use of services. The immediate circumstances in which a person feels unwell and makes (or does not make) the decision to consult or not to consult a doctor play an important part in their decision-making (Zola 1978; Robinson 1971; Finlayson and McEwen 1977; Salzberger 1976), and there is a tendency for people to rationalize their past behaviour in the light of subsequent events (Cowie 1976). This discussion is based entirely on retrospective accounts of consultations with doctors and experiences in hospitals, and there is no independent source of data – such as doctors' records or out-patient registers – with which to verify what people said about their use of health services.

Stimson and Webb (1975) have warned that lay people have a tendency to exaggerate the importance of their own contribution to the interactions that take place between them and their doctors. They say that people describe themselves as generally more assertive and more active in their relationships with doctors than they really are, and suggest, therefore, that lay accounts of medical consultations are best interpreted as reactions to relationships in which people feel (and often are made to feel) inferior, rather than accurate records of what in fact takes place between patients and doctors. This chapter does not ignore their warning but it does adopt a different approach to the accounts that people in this study gave of their experience as patients. As in previous chapters, this chapter distinguishes between the public and the private in the accounts of doctors and health services in the interviews. The public accounts tended to occur in answers to questions which were put to people directly about doctors and health services, such as:

What is your image of a 'good' doctor?
Did you attend ante-natal clinics when you were pregnant?
If Yes, why?
If No, why not?
How easy do you find talking to your doctor?

The private accounts were usually contained in the narrative of episodes which involved doctors but in which the doctors' activities were not the focus of attention.

In contrast to the situation Stimson and Webb describe, where – faced with an audience – their respondents became highly critical of doctors and told stories in which they personally appeared to get the better of doctors, the public accounts of doctors in the interviews were generally complimentary and markedly deferential and respectful of doctors and the medical profession. It was only in private accounts that people tended to be at all critical or derogatory about doctors, and even then the criticism was usually specific, i.e., it referred to one doctor in particular rather than to doctors in general.

It may be that the explanation for the different findings in the two studies is simply that they involve different groups of people with perhaps dissimilar experiences as patients. However, it is worth noting that the research methods employed in the two studies are different. Stimson and Webb interviewed respondents on their own but they also brought them together to discuss doctors in groups, and it was mostly in the groups that they observed people 'showing off' about getting the better of their doctors. That situation is entirely different from the one reported here, where the 'audience' consisted of (usually) no more than one other person – the interviewer. The attitudes Stimson and Webb report are as much products of the group situation and the group dynamic as public and private accounts are products of the research interviews. It seems likely that the effect of the group on the people taking part in it was to *legitimize* the content of what would otherwise have remained private accounts. In other words, the group made private accounts acceptable and in doing so created a new public account. If this is what happened, there is no reason to suppose that what people in the groups were saying was any more or less truthful than the public accounts in the interviews for this study. On the contrary, it would have been as partial and one-sided as all public accounts.

Whatever the explanation for the different findings in the two studies, the public accounts of doctors and health services in the interviews reported here pursued a limited set of themes. The attitude expressed towards doctors and towards medicine generally was admiring and respectful. Statements such as 'doctors are a breed, a certain breed of person' and 'all doctors are good doctors', were typical:

'To me, doctors and even nurses, this is something you do [offer respect]. I do, because to me they're doing a job I could never do and therefore I look up to them. I'm not saying they're all perfect but I still look up to them.'

Attitudes like these were based on the assumption that doctors are highly trained, scientific and technical workers who know things that ordinary people do not know. People repeatedly drew attention to the length of time it takes to become a doctor, to the fact that doctors have to study and learn from books and that being a doctor requires qualifications. However, the content of the public accounts varied with respect to different parts of the health service, and a hierarchy was erected in which hospital doctors were considered superior to general practitioners and both were considered superior to the medical staff of community health and preventive health clinics. The attitudes towards hospital doctors and hospital medicine (in general and acute hospitals rather than long-stay institutions for the mentally ill, chronic sick, and handicapped or disabled) were the most complimentary and respectful; the attitudes towards GPs were less complimentary and slightly critical; and the attitudes towards maternity and community health services were blatantly critical and openly sceptical about the usefulness of such services.

In contrast to the largely uniform and predictable content of public accounts, the private accounts of doctors and health services in the interviews were idiosyncratic and displayed attitudes towards medicine and the medical profession that were often complex and frequently contradictory. The impression they convey is one of immense variety in the experience of being a patient in the health service in East London, depending on the individual doctors and hospital departments involved in the care of the patient and on the nature of the problem that brought the patient into contact with them. Many, but by no means all, of the private accounts report experiences which from the point of view of the patient were unsatisfactory, and often the reason given was that the care received had been inexpert – in other words, the doctor had not known enough. The emotions aroused by doctors and health services reported in the private accounts were also far from straightforward. For example, the same person (Kathleen Read) said at one moment that she had absolute faith and confidence in a doctor who had treated her at a particular hospital, but later said it was right for her and other patients to be wary of all doctors because they can use their patients as 'guinea pigs' to experiment with new medical techniques.

This chapter describes the content of the different accounts of doctors and health services in the interviews and attempts to explain the discrepancies between them. It argues that both the public and the private accounts are products of medicalization; i.e., the attitudes and values they express are determined by the level or stage that has been reached in the interaction between modern, scientific (medical) legitimations for health and illness on the one hand, and traditional, normative (commonsense) legitimations on the other. The discrepancy betwen the two types of account indicates the overall significance and authority of medical legitimations for health and illness, as argued in previous chapters.

The discussion which follows is divided into three main sections. The first describes the background to the experiences reported in the interviews by giving a brief outline of the state of the health service in East London. The second and third sections present the content of the two types of account of doctors and health services in the interviews and explain the relevance of the concept of medicalization to them.

The local health service

The character of the health service in East London is both distinctive and unusual. It combines some of the most specialized and advanced medical services to be found anywhere with some of the most backward and under-developed community services, including general practice. In many ways it seems like a caricature of the National Health Service, in which the best and the worst have been grotesquely exaggerated.

Before the National Health Service was established, British medicine was already divided hierarchically between the hospital service and general practice (Honigsbaum 1979; Stevens 1966). The National Health Service confirmed this division and made it more pronounced. The separate contracts which the government negotiated with the general practitioners and the hospital consultants – in which general practitioners remained self-employed and contracted into the service whilst hospital doctors became salaried employees of the service – meant that general practice remained under-financed during a period in which the state took on the financial obligations of the hospital when capital investment was badly needed in the more advanced specialties. As a result, the hospital sector expanded whilst general practice – where investments in new facilities, equipment, or staff remained the GPs' private responsibility – remained under-developed and under-staffed (British Medical Association 1970; Royal College of General Practitioners 1977).

Thus in the first twenty years of the National Health Service the more prestigious positions within the medical profession continued to be in hospital medicine. The status attached to hospital medicine attracted applicants with better examination results and with degrees from Oxford and Cambridge and the more prestigious medical schools. The superior standards of treatment and care in hospitals, and especially in the teaching hospitals, in turn contributed to the greater prestige of hospital medicine. In general practice the opposite was happening. The medical students entering general practice tended to be those with poorer academic records who came from the less prestigious medical schools. General practice attracted the less qualified and the less motivated applicants and they, in turn, did little to arrest deteriorating standards and demoralization in this part of the health service (BMA 1970; RCGP 1977).

In the past ten to fifteen years the relationship between the two sides of the division in British medicine has begun to change. Publicly there had been growing disquiet about the relative costs and benefits of high technology medicine and this has coincided with cut-backs in public expenditure which have been directed at the health service, and at the hospital sector in particular. Medical students can no longer look forward to a safe career in hospital medicine simply because they have good examination results and, significantly, general practice is now the most popular career choice amongst medical students (RCGP 1977). At the same time, the foundation of the Royal College of General Practitioners (1967) and Michael Balint's work developing the necessary theoretical base for general practice to be able to lay claim to 'specialty' status have done much to improve the status of general practice within the medical profession (Armstrong 1979).

The relationship between the state and the medical profession and the part the state plays in determining the shape of the National Health Service is also changing. Since the mid-nineteen seventies the state has taken a more active role in the management of the service, establishing financial controls, introducing planning, and at the same time attempting to develop a national health policy (DHSS 1976a; 1976b; 1976c; 1979). The trend of government policy has been towards making the provision of services more equitable, between geographical regions and between the different sectors within the service. The *Report of the Resource Allocation Working Party* (DHSS 1976a) proposed a re-allocation of expenditure between the different geographical regions on the basis of a numerical assessment of health-care needs. Money was to be taken away from regions that had been particularly well funded and given to regions that were under-funded. At the same time, in *Priorities for Health and Social Service* (DHSS 1976b), the proposal was made to redistribute expenditure between the different parts of the service, so that money would be taken away from the acute medical services and used to develop community-based and preventive services and to improve care for the chronically ill.

General practitioners are not subject to direct control by the local or regional health authorities and this has meant that primary care has not been included in the redistribution of expenditure between the different parts of the health service. Psychologically, however, the impact of the policy has been considerable and has contributed to the re-ordering of the relationship between the divisions in British medicine. The recent emphasis on preventive health care and health promotion (DHSS 1979) has also helped to tip the balance further in favour of primary and community care and away from the acute medical services.

The particular part of the East End dealt with in this study is the area which, under the administrative arrangements existing prior to the most recent reorganization of the health service in 1982, was covered by two of the three District Health Authorities in the City and East London Area Health Authority (Teaching) – hereafter referred to as CELAHA(T): Tower Hamlets, and City and Hackney. The majority of people involved in the study live in Tower Hamlets District, and the remainder live in City and Hackney. The borders between the Districts are significant to local residents: as a general rule, the residents of Tower Hamlets think of the London Hospital (which has sites at Whitechapel and Mile End) as 'their' hospital, whilst the residents of Hackney see St Bartholomew's as more their own. There are also local hospitals with specialist functions and special reputations, such as the Queen Elizabeth Hospital for Children on Hackney Road (on the borders of the two Districts) and the London Chest Hospital in Bethnal Green, which everyone regardless of area of residence would think of using (see *Figure 2:1*, page 28).

The London Hospital and Bart's Hospital, both teaching hospitals with national and international reputations as 'centres of excellence' in medical teaching and research, are the biggest hospitals in CELAHA(T). Both contain specialist units funded by the North East Thames Regional Health Authority which are meant to service the entire population of the Region. Apart from the Regional specialties, both hospitals have individual doctors and specialist departments with reputations for excellence which attract patients from outside the immediate Districts, outside the Area, and sometimes outside the Region altogether. Thus in 1981, 73 per cent of patients in plastic surgery treated in Tower Hamlets came from outside the District and 10 per cent came from outside the Region altogether. Comparable figures for other specialties in Tower Hamlets show a similar pattern. Some, but not all, of these patients resident outside Tower Hamlets will be attending hospitals in Tower Hamlets from their places of work in the City and Central London.

Historically, both the London and Bart's have been exceptionally well endowed and have received a disproportionate share of the local health authority expenditure. In 1976, for example, acute medical services in Tower Hamlets received 73 per cent of the District health budget, which was a far greater proportion than that allocated to acute medical services nationally (55.5 per cent) (Yudkin 1978). The two sites at the London Hospital together account for the majority of acute medical beds and all the

Regional specialty beds in Tower Hamlets, and they received the greatest share of the money allocated to the acute medical services in the District. In 1978, according to Yudkin's (1978) estimates, the cost of the Regional specialty beds in the London Hospital to the District health authority was 20.8 per cent of the District's annual budget.

Both the teaching hospitals in CELAHA(T) survived relatively unscathed the rounds of cut-backs in spending on the health service initiated by the Labour government in the nineteen seventies. CELAHA(T) defended both hospitals vigorously against the redistributive policies proposed in RAWP (DHSS 1976a) and the '*Priorities*' document (DHSS 1976b), arguing that their exceptional status and financial privilages must be retained because as 'centres of special expertise' they constituted 'the heart of progress in British medicine' (CELAHA(T) 1976a: 1–2). Yudkin's analysis (1978) of resources in Tower Hamlets District following RAWP shows that whilst a 35 per cent reduction in acute beds which would reduce the amount actually spent on acute services by 13 per cent was projected for 1980–81, the hospital's *share* of the annual District budget was actually going to *increase* from 55.2 per cent spent in 1976 to 58.7 per cent in 1981. Cuts in spending would be made, but the teaching hospital would be cushioned from their worst effects; these would be borne by smaller hospitals in the District and by the community services.

In addition to the two teaching hospitals in CELAHA(T), Tower Hamlets and City and Hackney Health Districts have an unusual number of small hospitals providing acute services. Some, such as the Queen Elizabeth Hospital for Children, the Chest Hospital, and Moorfield's Eye Hospital, have specialized functions. The hospitals are not used exclusively by local residents but local residents account for a substantial proportion of their patients. For example, 58 per cent of the patients at Queen Elizabeth Hospital and 43 per cent of patients at the Chest Hospital are local residents (CELAHA(T) 1976a). Other hospitals, such as the London Jewish, the German Hospital, and Mildmay Mission, as the names indicate, either cater for a specific group of patients or were established in the tradition of missionary and charitable works in East London. The remaining hospitals, such as St Leonard's, Poplar Hospital, the Metropolitan, Bethnal Green, and others, are general hospitals serving relatively isolated communities. The suggestion that populations living so close to the City and to Central London are isolated may sound implausible, but public transport within the area is poor and often it is easier to travel into the City than it is to move relatively short distances within the two Districts.

Since the mid-nineteen seventies, many of the smaller hospitals have been closed down, and the ones that remain open do so under threat of closure or of conversion to some other use. Once it has been suggested that a hospital will be closed, it begins to run down. The fabric of the hospital is less well maintained, it becomes difficult to recruit or to keep staff and the existing staff become demoralized and therefore provide a lower quality of service. The threat of closure thus creates the conditions which are subsequently put forward to legitimate the hospital being closed (the hospital is too old; under-staffed; offers an inferior service; and so on). Standards of treatment and care in the hospitals inevitably deteriorate and, in comparison with the local teaching hospitals, the service is definitely second-rate.

The standard of primary health care in East London is generally recognised as being amongst the lowest in the country (Knox 1979). There is no shortage of doctors in the area. Recent figures for list sizes are not available but in 1974 there were 295 general practitioners in CELAHA(T) with average list sizes smaller than the national average (2,500). In 1983 there were 86 GPs in Tower Hamlets (personal communication from City and East London Family Practitioner Committee). The problem lies not with a shortage of doctors but with their methods and style of practice. In 1974, the proportion of GPs in the area who were in their sixties or older was almost twice the national average (27 per cent as opposed to 14 per cent); in the past nine years the figure has dropped to 22 per cent, of whom almost half are over seventy (City and East London FPC). This means that almost a quarter of the local GPs were recruited into general practice at the time when the status of general practice within the medical profession was exceptionally low.

Almost a quarter of GPs in Tower Hamlets (22 per cent) are in single-handed practice, and another quarter (24 per cent) in two-handed practice. This means that at least half the GPs in the District will not be able to provide a complete emergency service and will be reliant on medical deputies to make home visits and emergency calls at night. The majority of the GPs live outside the area and come into it only to work. One of the problems with primary health care locally, from the health authority's point of view, is that local residents use Accident and Emergency departments in hospitals for conditions that elsewhere would be treated in the community. The Authority believes that this unusual use of Accident and Emergency Services is connected to the standard of primary health care available locally. An internal enquiry into the work of the Accident and Emergency departments commissioned by CELAHA(T) in 1976 reported that:

'The tradition of visiting the hospital casualty department rather than the general practitioner remains but might be appreciably altered if the casual patients knew that their own primary care teams were adequately accommodated and equipped to provide the service.' (1976b: 3)

In 1983, there were four purpose-built health centres in Tower Hamlets (City and East London FPC); the vast majority of the local GPs work from premises that are converted shops or terraced houses. Most have no space to accommodate other workers and do not operate as members of a primary health care team including district nurses, health visitors, chiropodists, receptionists, and social workers. The situation is made worse by under-staffing in the community services. Recent figures were not obtained for levels of staffing in the community health services, but in 1975 CELAHA(T) reported shortages of health visitors, school nurses, and chiropodists, and envisaged that these would become worse rather than better in the years to come.

The characteristics of the physical and social environment in East London make it unattractive to professional health workers, and to doctors especially. Within the medical profession, general practice in exclusively working-class areas is considered unglamorous and unrewarding (Cartwright 1967; Knox 1979), and time spent in practice in such areas is seen as 'almost certain disqualification for any further career advancement' (Knox 1979: 115; Tudor Hart 1971). Not surprisingly, therefore, it is difficult to recruit doctors and other health professionals into East London, and in 1974 CELAHA(T) envisaged 'serious shortages' in medical manpower in primary care as well as the community services, developing over the next ten to fifteen years (CELAHA(T) 1975). The new posts which do fall vacant, as is typical in inner city areas (Knox 1979) are increasingly filled by doctors, often from overseas, who find it difficult to get jobs in other parts of the health service.

Public accounts of doctors and health services

The health service, which has been described above, is the one that people in the study know, the one in which they are patients. Their attitudes towards doctors and health services, as expressed in public accounts in the interviews, are based on certain assumptions about the nature of medicine and medical practice. The principal assumption, and the one that gives rise to the host of meanings they associate with doctors and health services, is that medicine is *a science*. If medicine is scientific, to them this means: (i) medical practitioners are superior to ordinary people because they know more, are more intelligent and more advanced in learning than ordinary people; (ii) it requires dedication and self-sacrifice to become a doctor, and it is right to respect doctors for this; (iii) the object of medical science – the health problems which doctors treat – is extra-ordinary in the sense of being beyond the powers of ordinary people to treat and requiring specialized knowledge; and (iv) the implications of the previous points are that medicine and the medical profession are not to be taken lightly. The proper object of medical attention is serious illness and it is not right for doctors to have to be bothered with health problems that people can treat themselves or with 'trivial' problems.

In the interviews, most of the definitions of medical work, and many of the respondents' descriptions of the medical profession, were given in the context of comparisons between medicine and social work. The term 'social work' was used indiscriminately to mean probation officers, almoners, the medical and nursing staff of mother and baby and child health clinics, health visitors, and district nurses as well as social workers employed by local social services. The medical and nursing staff mentioned were also frequently referred to as 'welfare workers'. The purpose of these comparisons was to demonstrate the extra-ordinariness of medicine as opposed to the ordinariness of commonsense, with social work being the epitome of commonsense. Commonsense, in these terms, meant the knowledge that ordinary people have that comes from their life-experience. Thus medical knowledge and medical skills were said to be appropriate to problems that ordinary people cannot cope with, whereas commonsense was said to be what was required to deal with the ordinary problems of everyday life, i.e., those that they see tackled by social workers.

The comparisons between medicine and social work in public

accounts invariably followed the same lines of argument. People drew attention to the training required to become a doctor, and especially to the book-learning involved, contrasting this with the supposed lack of training and book-learning required to become a social worker:

'[Doctors] have had to go through tests and all that. They've had to learn something to do their sort of job. Social workers, nine times out of ten anyone could do it. [If I go to the doctor] I'm hoping he's done his job properly and he's learned his job, his skills, and he knows what he's talking about. If I go to him in great pain, I'm hoping when I go up there that he can tell me what is wrong with me. I don't want him turning round and saying to me, "Well, it could be this or it could be that". Then I think to myself, "You're a doctor. You went through all that rigmarole of learning. Surely you could tell me what this pain is." But a social worker, I think it's just a job anyone can do, anyone with commonsense.'

If people in the study had any (direct) involvement with social workers, it was usually on account of their relationship to their children. Kathleen Read, Joe Hutchinson, Mick Chalmers, and Joanne Goode had, for various reasons, all had dealings with social workers, and it is perhaps worthy of notice that in each case it had been in the period of their lives when they were living as single parents. Joanne distinguished between doctors and social workers on grounds that the problems they dealt with were different: medical problems were 'objective' whilst social work problems were 'subjective', meaning idiosyncratic and personal:

'I think the welfare people and things like that are dealing with more delicate things. It's – they're dealing with personal, they're not dealing with medical . . . I don't feel I could treat the two on the same basis because with the medical you are not actually being given advice, you're being given treatment. But when it comes to welfare and social workers, they are giving you advice, they're not giving you treatment. They're giving you advice which half the time they probably haven't had experience of themself. And as soon as – all people are individual – I mean, when you look at medicine, cancer is cancer no matter who it's in. All right, it might be cancer, if it's cancer of the lung it might be in six different men. But when you have a woman having problems with her child, them problems are different for each individual woman because each woman is an individual, she is different. So that is where they differ for a start. The fact that a cancer is a cancer no matter whose body it's in, but a problem is an individual thing because of the person being an individual. So I don't see how they can block it down, either you remove or you cure or whatever. It is a thing. But with a problem, you might have a problem but you might treat it in a different way to what I would, even if it's the same problem. So I don't see how you can advise people, not by going from books and exams and things like that.'

The meanings people associated with medicine and social work determined their expectations and their criticisms of doctors and social workers respectively. Most people said that the doctor's personality and his manner (doctors were always, collectively, male) were less important than that he should know what he was doing and should be good at his job. There was a noticeable difference in the attitudes of people in different generations in this respect, although it was not great. The older people in the study had affection as well as respect for the doctors they remembered from before the past war. The difference between their attitudes and the attitudes of the younger people can be best expressed as the difference between a simple class respect – the older people respected doctors as socially superior beings – and a respect for academic and technical qualifications.

Kathleen Read had a greater history of involvement with doctors than anybody else in the group. Her idea of a 'good doctor' was one who could make her better, and she said she was not bothered by whether or not they had a good bedside manner. In her view the best doctors who had treated her – one at the Chest Hospital and one a previous GP – had also been the rudest and the most aggressive:

'As long as they can do their job, as far as I'm concerned, I mean . . . someone, as far as I know, who can do his job and can take what's wrong with me and put it right . . . They can be aggressive, they can be sympathetic. Sometimes I think sympathetic people make you weepy anyway if they sympathize with you, if they feel sorry for you. I don't think it does any good, to be honest. You've got to have someone, that's going to make you fight to get well.'

The order of priorities people stated most frequently with

reference to doctors is summed up in the following passage in which Ann Cullen distinguishes between the 'main thing' and the added extra which would 'be nice':

'The main thing, I think, with a good doctor, is to know what he's doing of. And another thing I think, if you've got this doctor and you're going to have him for years, it's nice to be able to talk to him, if you've got one of the doctors and you can talk to them and they'll listen to you. But a lot of them don't.'

Ann went on to excuse doctors for being short with their patients on the grounds that 'their time is vital to them, naturally' and 'they've got such a lot to do':

'They can't afford to sit and talk to me for an hour or nothing like this. But what I'm trying to say is, if I go to my doctor and I'm worried about something and I say to him that I'm worried, as long as he's got the time to say to me, "No, that's nothing to worry about", that's fair enough. But you do get some doctors and "Oh, that's nothing to worry about", and they haven't even got the time to talk to you. I'm not saying they don't want to talk to you, they haven't always got the time to talk to you because they have got so many patients and there's so much to do that their time is valuable.'

Other people, and especially the younger people, were less charitable than Ann, and more overtly critical of doctors who gave the impression of having no interest in their patients:

'You go into them and so many people go into the doctor, in the end you're just a number. He don't see the faces in the end, I don't think. So he talks to you and he reads the notes and he ends up not actually seeing you.'

'All you do is go in there and all they do is keep writing and grunting. Don't say nothing to you. And you've got to keep making yourself look an idiot and keep saying, "Well, what about so and so? Is that all right?" "Mm." "Well, what about that?" "Mm." And that's all you get. I know it's probably their time, they haven't got the time. But surely the time you take to go "Mm" is the time to say "Yes" or "No" or "No, it's all right". It can only take as much.'

Despite these complaints about doctors' manner, the main expectation that people in the study had of doctors was that they should do their job and should be seen by their patients to be doing their job, properly. Their most severe criticism was of doctors whom they judged inadequate in this respect. Thus, Mick Chalmers was damning about his previous GP:

'He was useless to me, he didn't give me no confidence at all. I thought to myself, "If I'm really ill, I wouldn't like to go to him because I don't think he'd be able to diagnose a pimple on the end of me nose". He gives me that impression. I think a doctor's better off, I think it makes a person feel better if they're ill and they go into the doctor's room and the doctor says, "Come and sit down", and he gives him the confidence that he knows what he's talking about and that he can help you.'

Ben Knight was thoroughly disappointed with his treatment as an out-patient, precisely because there was nothing to indicate to him that something positive was being done by the doctors responsible for his case:

'Now when I go to the hospital, the first thing they say is, "How are you feeling?". But there's no real test to see if my blood is in good order. I think they wait for you to fall down and then they turn round and say, "Oh, he's got something wrong there". And then they will see you. Although they looked after me well while I was in hospital – I suppose perhaps it might be – but I feel I'm wasting their time. To take time off work to go to the hospital and have them just tell me, "Are you all right? How do you feel?" I would sooner go to the doctor's and I want them to say, "It's your blood. Just test it. How do you feel? O.K. We'll see you in . . ." But when they ask questions and don't test nothing, it amazes me. It amazes me.'

The criteria people applied in their judgments of individual doctors involved three different aspects of medical work: diagnosis, physical examinations and tests, and prescriptions. With respect to all three, their image of the 'good doctor' conformed exactly with Balint's account of the orthodox style of medical practice thirty years ago which he calls 'elimination by appropriate physical examinations' (Balint 1957: 37–44). The sequence of steps taken by the doctor who operates in this style is as follows: the doctor enquires about the patient's symptoms; conducts a physical examination; makes a diagnosis; and prescribes treatment. If the patient does not improve, or if the doctor cannot make a diagnosis on the basis of his examination, the doctor refers the patient to a specialist and continues to refer him or her until a diagnosis is made and a successful course of treatment prescribed.

This is exactly the sequence of steps that people in the study expect their doctors to follow, and if they criticized their doctors at all, they criticized them for three things: failing to diagnose or making the wrong diagnosis; not making clinical examinations or doing clinical tests (this is consistent with Skrimshire's finding (1978) amongst patients in Newham); always ending the consulation with a prescription and prescribing the same medicine for different conditions (again, this is consistent with the findings in other studies where it is reported that patients do not want prescriptions as much as their doctors believe they do (Cartwright 1967; Stimson and Webb 1975).

In the past, everyone in the Davies family and all of Stan Flowers's relatives had been in the care of the same local GP, whose style of practice all of them admired. This doctor did not 'sit and chat' with his patients, he asked them their symptoms, conducted a physical examination, and told them what was wrong. He only prescribed a medicine if he felt it was necessary and often told his patients they must manage without drugs. If he did prescribe a medicine it was nearly always different from ones he prescribed on other occasions and this convinced his patients he knew what he was doing. This was in contrast with other doctors whom many people felt prescribed drugs regardless of what was wrong with the patient.

> 'They talk to you, but at the end they give you the same stuff, so what's the point of the chat? You know what the kids are going to get. I feel like saying, "Oh, don't bother, I've still got some indoors from last time". You know exactly what you're going to get for the kids and, as I say, it can only be aspirin-based or paracetomol or something like that. I mean, what's the point of going up there if you're going to get the same stuff all the time? Why not just say to the mother, "Well, just take them home and give them a couple of aspirins". That's probably why the NHS is in such bad shape. They just dish out these bottles of medicine. I think they just do it to keep you quiet.'

If the medicine the Davies's GP prescribed did not 'do the trick', as Kathleen put it, there were no 'second chances'. His patients knew they would be referred straight away to one of the local hospitals for further investigations, and again, this was something all of them approved of.

The attitudes towards social workers expressed in public accounts in the interviews were the exact opposite of those expressed towards doctors. When they were discussing social work and social workers, people made no attempt to choose their words carefully or to seem respectful towards social workers either as individuals or as a professional group. In contrast with the criteria they applied in their judgments of doctors, they said that the most important consideration with respect to social workers was what kind of person they were. The right people for social work, they felt, were women who were married and had children:

'Social workers, as I say, it's a pity they've got so many young ones. If they could get, like, mothers – a woman who's brought up her own family and has got more time on her hands, if she could – because it's not from, sometimes, reading out of books that helps, it's experience and you can deal with it better by how you brought up your children.'

In contrast with the criticisms of individual doctors for not doing their job properly, the criticisms of individual social workers were that they were the wrong sort of person:

'It was a young fella that turned up, and we didn't hit it off at all . . . And I turned round and said, "Well, you're a right one. What do you know about life", I says, "to try and say to me about bringing up kids? You don't look old enough to have any and you probably haven't." "Oh no." You know he wasn't even married or anything.'

'They was like old women, in their fifties. Miss This and Miss That, who've never had no bloody kids of their own, which to me was ridiculous. Because it's all right saying they've studied over years, but it's not the same as bringing them up yourself. They may have read so many books, but until you've looked after a child every day for so many months, you don't really know what it's like and how they get on your nerves.'

'She was a young girl and she was trying to tell me about kids and she wasn't even married or had any herself. She was telling me what she read out of books. And I don't think I wanted to be told by someone like that.'

The difference in the content of public accounts of doctors and social workers is based on the distinction between science and commonsense, and that distinction is also at the bottom of the different attitudes people had towards different parts of the health service. As we have seen, people in the study rank medicine superior to ordinary commonsense and doctors as more important than social workers (who are on a par with themselves and other ordinary folk) because medicine has to be learned and because it treats problems which are beyond the capabilities of the ordinary person to treat. When this frame of reference is applied to the health service they distinguish between its different parts according to the type of problem the service treats, specified in terms of the tri-partite classification of health problems outlined in Chapter 5. Thus the service for which they have the greatest respect is the hospital service because it deals with 'real' illness; GPs are positioned lower down the hierarchy because their province is, first and foremost, 'normal' illness, and to a lesser extent 'real' illness in the sense that they supply the referral to a specialist; at the bottom are the community services (school health; mother and baby clinics; child health clinics; health visiting) and the maternity services (ante-natal clinics and classes and the obstetric service), which deal with health problems which are not illness.

To a certain extent, the hierarchical approach to the health service accurately reflects people's experience of being patients in the local health service. They preferred large hospitals to small hospitals, and teaching hospitals to other hospitals, because they believed – with reason – that the staff in these hospitals were better trained and the hospitals were better equipped. William Cox, for example, had twice been treated for a knee injury, the first time in St Leonard's Hospital in Hackney, and the second time at the London Hospital, Whitechapel. At St Leonard's, he had a painful operation performed on his knee without local anaesthetic; at the London the same operation was performed with a local anaesthetic. On the basis of this experience, William and his family had concluded that the London is the better hospital of the two and had generalized this observation to all teaching hospitals and to larger as opposed to smaller hospitals.

The idea that general practice is less prestigious and less important than hospital medicine is confirmed for many people by the shabbiness of many of the local surgeries and by the difficulty they have in seeing the doctor. This is how Kathleen Read described the difference in her feelings in anticipation of a visit to the local surgery compared with a visit to an out-patient clinic in hospital:

'If it's just an ordinary GP now, I hardly have to go up there, I only have to go for me tablets, I take no notice. But if it's to go to the hospital for anything or other, although you've got confidence in them, I still get awful butterflies. Although I'm discharged from the Chest Hospital, I can ring them up for an appointment on that morning, although I know everybody up there I still feel sick as a dog. I can't eat, which is ridiculous really, I suppose, unless it might be fear of the outcome of what you're going up there for, I don't know. But the actual doctors and that, I still get the colly wobbles, hospital-wise anyway, not so much me GP.'

Many of the complaints people had about the practical arrangements in their local practice are consistent with the description of general practice in East London above. The most common complaint was that local GPs do not work an appointment system, but see their patients instead on the basis of first come, first served. For patients this can mean waiting anything from a few minutes to a couple of hours to see the doctor and not being able to predict in advance which it will be, something which is especially irksome for women with young children. People complained that the waiting rooms were also often uncomfortable and unpleasant, and said they were afraid of catching something while they waited to see the doctor.

The complaints about some of the community and maternity services were very similar to the complaints about general practice. The women (for it is women who use these services in the main) complained that it was difficult to get appointments at the Family Planning Clinics and they were kept waiting for long periods at ante-natal clinics. Underlying their complaints was the feeling that the staff who ran the clinics were not interested in their patients. This was Sharon Berthot's description of her visits to the ante-natal clinic at the London Hospital:

'I hated it. You sit up there for hours, four hours sometimes we'd be up there at the London. You'd get up there at quarter to one, by five o'clock you're just walking out of the place.'
JC: 'What did they do to you in the clinic?'
'Not a lot, waiting time really. I mean by the time you, all right you had your blood pressure taken, you used to have to give a urine sample, you was weighed. The actual time that you spent with the doctors must have been five minutes. So I mean you had about ten minutes actually doing anything, and all the rest

was waiting time. I can understand why people don't go. All those mothers crammed together into a little space, all waiting to do the same thing. Oh, it was horrible.'

JC: 'Did you get anything out of going to the clinic? Did you talk to the doctor, or ask questions?'

'He didn't seem to have time, to be honest. I mean, they'd come in and they'd say, "Oh, yes, Mrs Berthot, how are you?" and you'd go, "Uh". "Yes, well you're doing fine, we'll see you in a fortnight's time." "Yeah, yeah – I'm fine." It was like that. They really didn't have the time. I suppose if there was anything really wrong with you, you'd push it. But I suppose, I mean they've just had so many cases of morning sickness and feeling dizzy that they just don't want to know anymore. That's the way I found it.'

Some complaints were harder to unravel. For example, Jackie Cox combined her resentment of the care (or lack of it) received at the mother and baby clinic with her prejudice against the local Bengali population. Nevertheless, the basic message, which was her dissatisfaction with the clinic, was the same:

'Them babies [meaning the Bengali babies], I mean they [the clinic staff] had the cheek to turn round and say to me about putting her on solids when there was a dear little Pakistani baby in there and it had a tea-towel for a nappy, and I wouldn't have put that tea-towel in my dog's basket, let alone a baby's bum. And they have the cheek to tell me off and let that poor little baby lay there. The clothes it had was filthy, and it was dirty, and they're sort of saying to her, "Very good, very good". Not saying nothing. And they come out and what done me in, I had a row up there and wouldn't go in there, and they come out and went all along to the Pakistanis sitting there and they went, "Here you are. There's free samples of Milupa food." Well, that's what I give her, the puddings, powdered stuff. Well it's dear, eighty pence a box. "There you are, for baby, baby's food." All, give them out, all of them, and left me out. My mate said to me, "You use that stuff, don't you?". I said, "Yes, I do". And you don't get it because they think you. And them babies, some of them are as old as her and they look like little rats, honestly they had no flesh on them. And they turned round and said it was because they weren't giving them anything.'

It is clear that people's experience as patients in the local health services partially accounts for their attitudes towards different parts of the service, but it does not entirely explain them. For example, it does not adaquately explain their hostility towards the maternity services. Most of the ante-natal care they receive and the majority of their babies are delivered in hospitals, and in every other instance they are respectful of hospital medicine. It also does not explain the pattern of their generalizing: they generalize from individual examples of 'bad' social workers, 'bad' nurses, and doctors in community clinics and poor service in ante-natal and obstetrics to the service as a whole, but they do not generalize from cases of individually 'bad' hospital doctors to hospital medicine.

A possible explanation for the hierarchy they apply to the different parts of the health service might be that they are so indoctrinated by the medical profession that they simply reproduce medical values and priorities. Without wishing to portray medicine or the medical profession as monolithic entities (Freidson 1970; Strong 1979a,b), this hypothesis seems both plausible and persuasive. The attitudes which were expressed in the interviews are perfectly compatible with those which – perhaps until very recently – were common amongst the more dominant sections of the medical profession, and are certainly consistent with the aspects of medicine that receive the most media attention. Again, however, the hypothesis is only partially adequate for it fails to account for the women's profound resistance to and rejection of the community and maternity services. The medical orthodoxy with respect to the maternity services – or the 'medical frame of reference' as Oakley (1980) calls it – advocates medical supervision of every stage of the reproductive process, from early pregnancy through to childbirth and post-natal care of the mother and infant. It does so on the grounds that early and regular attendance at ante-natal clinics, hospital deliveries, and the tuition of mothers in the care of the infant by medical and nursing staff, have been responsible for the decline in maternal and infant mortality (a claim endorsed by the Department of Health (DHSS 1976c).

The women in this study do not share this view. They regard the different stages of the reproductive process as potential health problems but not illness, and in their view the proper way to manage them is by learning from experience (one's own and other women's) and using commonsense. They believe that the experience of childbirth is different for each woman and varies from one pregnancy to the next, which makes it impossible for anyone else to instruct them in how to cope with it. Only two of the women – Sharon and Jackie – attended relaxation classes before they had their first baby, and in both their cases something unusual happened during their labour. Sharon's baby was delivered unusually quickly, and Jackie's turned into an emergency when the baby showed signs of distress. Both women felt the classes were of no help in coping with what had happened, neither went back to the classes with subsequent pregnancies and neither would recommend the classes to other women:

> 'So there's me, sitting and taking it all in and, as it turned out, it just didn't happen that way. I mean, they tell you it does take a long time, your first baby and all this, and not to go to the hospital too soon because you won't be very pleased by waiting hours in the hospital. And at first you'll just have these niggly pains, maybe a back ache, then you'll have a show and then they said like, just get prepared for it. Get your suitcase ready and potter about indoors. When the time comes, like, say they're coming every twenty minutes, then go to the hospital. Fine, fine. They didn't tell me it could go completely wrong and sometimes it just doesn't happen that way. They don't tell you that. So there's me waiting for them to come every twenty minutes and the poor little sod was nearly born in me mother's bed.'

We know from the discussion of relationships between female relatives in Chapter 4 that most of the women had not talked to their mothers or sisters about childbirth and were often totally unprepared for their first experience of it. However, once they had one baby, in their view they were as knowledgeable about the whole process as anyone else; certainly as knowledgeable as the medical and nursing staff who delivered their subsequent babies. It is significant therefore that seven out of the ten women in the study with more than one child described head-on clashes with the staff during the delivery of babies other than their first born:

> 'I know it's different, isn't it, after you've had the first one. You know the second time what's going on. So I woke Paul up and we got to the hospital about six o'clock. Of course I walked in, I says, "Oh, here's me card". She goes, "You're not in strong labour yet, you can have a bath". I says, "I ain't getting in a

bath, I'm going to have it soon". "No, no, you've got plenty of time." You know, they won't listen. I said, "No. I know that it's going to happen fast." And of course by the time I go into what they call strong labour at six-fifteen and she was born at six-thirty. And the doctor wasn't even there because she hadn't called him. She'd run a bath and was expecting me to get into the bath.'

'I was in for bed rest and I started getting pains in me back, and I thought, this is it. So I called up the nurse and she said "Come up here", she said, "you're only in for bed rest". "I don't care what I'm in here for", I said, "my pains have started". So she gave me an injection. She said I'd be all right after a sleep. So that was like on the Saturday night and I had a little couple of hours kip and something woke me up again. I rang the bell again. "Nurse", I said, "they definitely are labour pains I'm getting in me back". "No", she said, "you're not down to have him yet". I said, "I ain't got a date for when". And the girl in the next bed said, "Oh, isn't it ridiculous. You'd think they'd take you down there and get you prepared." And about, what was it? Half past seven, I held on to that bell. I said, "If you don't hurry and get me down there I'll have it in this bed". "Oh, my God", she said, "the head's there", and the next thing it was like panic stations.'

These were the only situations described in public accounts of health services in the interviews in which anyone – man or woman – said that they knew better than the medical staff, and although there were other situations in which people described themselves having arguments with medical staff, these were the only occasions on which it was the patient who did the arguing. At other times it was a relative of the patient who was said to have tackled the doctor, usually after the incident in question had blown over. The justification the women gave for their behaviour was the same justification they gave for their attitudes towards social workers. To them, the knowledge that was required in this particular situation was commonsense knowledge based on personal experience. They expected the staff to be the 'right sort of person', and did not expect to be told what to do by them:

'I never went to the classes, so I never found out if the women who give the classes have ever had children to sort of. Now, now that would be a thing. If the woman's sitting there and she's never had kids and turns round and says to me, "Now, if you do this it'll be easier". Then I would actually turn round and say, "Well, how the hell do you know if you've never had a baby?". "Do you know that it's going to make it easier?" They can only go by what they're told and by advice.'

'Like they say to you "pant" and all that. To me, that's a load of old codswallop. Panting and stop. All right, I know they need to see if the cord's round the baby's neck and all that. But when I had Lynne, they used to say "Stop. Pant" [her voice stern and authoritarian]. I just used to bear down, didn't I? All this bleeding . . . More pain for me. So, I don't know. Maybe some people need to do it and all that. But once the head is through, then the baby just comes away anyway.'

The women's attitudes towards child health and mother and baby clinics was much the same. They felt that what the service and the clinics offered was basically commonsense advice on how to look after a child. The only people in need of such a service were women who did not have mothers or sisters who could tell them what to do. Peggy Freeman and Sarah Chalmers had been living too far away from their families when they had their first child for their mothers to have been much practical use, and both of them said they had valued their contact with health visitors and clinic staff. However, as Peggy pointed out, she had not returned to the clinics with her second baby:

'More so the first one, I think, but I didn't bother much with Ron [the second baby], because you're more experienced and you know what you're doing of and you don't really need to take them along to the clinic. Pick something up, I always think. I always got the feeling that they might come up with measles, go in fit and pick up a germ. So I didn't bother much with the second one, only when it was injection time I'd take them.'

The other women felt that health visitors and the clinics were there to deal with 'special cases', an identity they rejected for themselves especially because, in common with the women in Aberdeen whom Blaxter and Paterson interviewed (1982), they strongly believed that the principal function of the clinics was to identify battered babies and children:

'For some people they are probably very good things, especially for those girls who are not married and whose mothers don't want to know. They're the people who are there to help them and to ask questions, which is a good thing. But if you've got.

Let me put it this way. Like my Jackie, she's got all of us and whatever. I'm not saying she don't need them, but what I'm trying to say is, it's not so necessary for her to go as a girl would who was on her own. Whose mothers perhaps said, "Well, you got into trouble, and you've got to get on with it". Which do happen . . . So I think that these people are needed, if not by my Jackie, by thousands of others and I think it's a good thing to have them. And I think it's a good thing for them to be there because if some of these girls do go they can see if the baby's being neglected. For the child's sake alone I think they should be there.'

One of the mechanisms that contributes to the dominance of medicine and of modern (scientific) legitimations in the process of medicalization is the impact that medical and scientific achievements make on people's consciousness. Some comments in the interviews show how the process works. Mary Webb's attitudes towards doctors and social workers and towards the different parts of the health service were consistent with the attitudes outlined above *except* that she had a passionate belief in the importance of ante-natal care for pregnant women. She had attended ante-natal clinics regularly during all of her pregnancies and insisted that her daughter follow her example. The reason for this was that Mary knew from her own experience about complications in pregnancy which could be avoided with proper ante-natal supervision:

'Like me with . . . If I hadn't gone, they wouldn't have known that I had this toxaemia and all the rest of it, so it was a good thing I did go. I used to, as I say, I was in hospital a month before Steven was born, but you don't realise what a killer that can be for the unborn child. Not so much the mother, is it? It's the unborn child it affects more than it does the mother.'

Ann Cullen also approved of ante-natal care and she too gave specific medical reasons for why she thought it was a good thing:

'Let's be fair, pregnancy – to me – blood pressure, you've got to be very careful of, and that must be worth going for on its own, to make sure you have your blood pressure checked to make sure that it is normal. I mean, in pregnancy, if you've got high blood pressure, it can turn into toxaemia.'
JC: 'Does than mean you encouraged Jackie to go?'
'Oh yes, because I think it is right. I think you should go. I mean, they take your water when you do go, and they take

your blood pressure and they take blood every so often, which is a good thing. At least they know if things are going wrong, they can tell by this and they can take you in and do a lot of things. Whereas, if you're not going and it happens, you can't blame anybody else but yourself, can you? Let's be fair.'

The difference between Mary and Ann and the other women suggests something about how the process of medicalization works. Nevertheless, the point we return to in commenting on public accounts of doctors and health services in general, is the significance of the images of medical practice and the medical profession which dominate them. The interviews show that the images dominate the ideological framework within which people make sense of their experience to such an extent that where there is a discrepancy between the two, the experience and not the image is made redundant (the positive image of the medical profession overrides memories of 'bad' doctors, wrong diagnoses, prescriptions that are unwanted and do not work, to make 'all doctors', in hospital and in general practice, 'good doctors'). This point can be made more forcibly by comparing the descriptions of doctors and health services in public and private accounts, as we do below. The level that medicalization of the ideological framework had reached was high enough to ensure that, most of the time, the public accounts people gave recreated and reproduced images of medicine that bore no necessary relationship to their personal experience. The exceptions were the community and maternity services where they appealed to personal experience to legitimate equally partial and one-sided public accounts.

Private accounts of doctors and health services

It is much less easy to identify common themes in private accounts of doctors and health services than in public accounts. The private accounts in the interviews consist mostly of stories about how a particular doctor, hospital department, or hospital ward behaved on a particular occasion, and they were very varied. For example, they included stories of:

– people who radically altered their opinion of their GP in the course of a relationship which lasted many years. Joe Hutchinson was one of these people. His relationship with his GP had begun with him having a low opinion of the doctor as a result of the GP's casual treatment of the family. Joe had felt that the doctor had been uninterested in Joe's wife when she had breast cancer, and had developed a great antipathy towards him after the doctor had refused to call at the house when Joe's father suffered a stroke during the Easter holiday period. Later, however, when Joe was a widower bringing up four young children as a single parent, he had found the GP considerate and supportive, and he had begun to like him.

- the same person having different attitudes towards different doctors. This was common in the group. Kathleen Read, for example, had liked and respected the doctor referred to earlier who had cared for most of her relatives, but her opinion of her present GP was low. Ann Cullen liked the woman doctor in the group practice she attended, but refused to see one of the other doctors after she had a row with him (described in brief below). Jeannie Moss liked two out of the three doctors in her group practice but avoided appointments with the third.

- different people having different attitudes towards the same doctor. Thus the GP whom Kathleen Read disliked, Ben Knight admired and respected.

Although the private accounts contain a mass of stories which tell of highly varied reactions and responses on the part of this group of people to their doctors and to health services, the theme of doctors' power, and of the social distance between doctors and patients created by it, is constant. It is not appropriate to repeat all the stories but by concentrating on the variety of responses to the phenomenon of medical power/authority, one hopes to give an impression of their range and diversity. The stories which have been selected tend to describe poor experiences of being a patient because in private accounts these were the stories that were more frequent.

It has been suggested already that people in the group had more respect for hospital medicine than general practice. This was borne out in the private accounts which showed that they experienced medical power and authority much more intensely in hospital settings. Kathleen is quoted above as being more nervous about hospital appointments than she is of seeing her GP, and this was a feeling that other people shared with her. The impression the private accounts give of events in hospital is that of events that take place on a grand scale. If a person feels well-treated by doctors in hospital, this goes down in their memory as something marvellous; if they are mistreated, or if their case is handled wrongly, their response – whether angry or disappointed – is equally exaggerated. Thus Sharon Berthot remembered appreciatively the doctors who had treated her father in hospital when he was dying from lung cancer fifteen years previously:

'He'd say, "How much homework have you got tonight?", you know, like, "What are you doing? What subjects are you doing at school?" And I felt more – that the doctor cared about you as well, the way you was feeling, the way you was taking everything. Not like – oh, you know – "Your father's dying and that's the end of it, you've got to go away and cope on your own". They seemed concerned for the whole family, like they know that they're dealing with a sick man, but they seemed concerned about what effect it's having on the family as well. Not just one person. Which is something I never really considered, doctors being that way.'

On the other hand, Betty Mayes and Kathleen Read (amongst others) both told stories about incidents where they felt a hospital doctor had not done his job properly, for which they held them completely and personally responsible. Both women felt bitterly angry about these incidents; feelings that were in direct proportion to the magnitude of their expectations that these doctors should have known everything and should not have made mistakes.

The story Betty Mayes told was of a doctor at Bethnal Green Hospital who had failed to diagnose her mother's breast cancer. When the diagnosis was made (at the London Hospital, thus confirming the belief that teaching hospitals are better than the small community hospitals), Betty had gone to the first doctor's out-patient clinic and accused him, in public, of killing her mother. After her mother died she went back to the clinic, called him a murderer and hit him with a heavy ashtray which was lying on the desk.

Kathleen's story was about the failure of gynaecologists at the London to diagnose her last pregnancy soon enough for it to be terminated:

'I'd definitely got the fibroids and that was all the others could feel was the fibroids. "Well, we'll send her down for a scan." So I goes for a scan. "Well, it might be and it might not be, I can't see a baby on the scan. I can only make out the fibroid." I said,

"Right, well go and tell Dr Williams", which is what the student's name was. And Dr Williams still insisted that I was pregnant. I thought, God Almighty, what's going to – what can you do to prove that I'm not, sort of thing. So he brings out this wireless contraption, all wires, just to prove he is right and all the others are wrong. And he went, plonk. He said, "That's the baby's heart". Well everyone was amazed. It's a wonder I didn't die of shock. "You're pregnant", he said, "so we can't do the operation". I said, "And whose fault is that? I've been coming up and down for three months", I said, "and everyone says I'm not", I said, "and if you'd proved it earlier I could have had the abortion done, couldn't I?" . . . So I turned round and said to Mr Weston, he said, "Well, we might as well discharge you and you can come back after the baby's born". I turned round and said, "Right, I'll go to the first back-street abortionist I can find". He said, "Even a back-street abortionist wouldn't touch you with the inside that you've got". So I thought, well what do I do? Come home and jump from the top of the stairs to the bottom? You know. Everyone consoled me and said wait and see, but I said, if there was a mark on her I'd never have brought her out [of the hospital] anyway.'

There are other stories, hints, and passing comments in private accounts which contribute to the picture of people in the study having a much greater sense of medical power and authority in hospitals. Ann Cullen, for example, never dared ask the doctors at the London Hospital what was wrong with her husband after he had suffered three strokes, but waited to find out from her GP (whom she knew hardly at all).

The tone of the stories about GPs in private accounts is much more muted than that of the stories about hospitals, but it was otherwise much the same. The personal reactions the stories describe are based on the premise that the doctor has more power than the patient and the relationship between them is therefore unequal. In some cases, the patient's response to that situation is to be assertive. Peggy Freeman, for example, had decided that she would dictate referrals to hospital for her family, and also decide which hospital they should go to. Stan Flowers was triumphant because he had been able to fool his doctor into providing him with the sick certificate he needed to claim benefits when he was put on short-time working. Mick Chalmers was defiant about having rejected to his face the advice his GP gave him. The point about such stories is that the person telling the story felt involved in an unequal contest. The emotions the doctors aroused were the product of their subordinate position. Thus, the following quotation from an interview with Ann Cullen shows how difficult it can be for the patient (or, in this case, a relative of the patient) to cope with the situation in which this powerful medical figure fails to live up to the patient's expectations. The doctor in the story had mis-diagnosed Eddie Cullen's first stroke as nerves, and told him to go home and rest. Later, when he appeared in response to an emergency call, Ann had refused to allow him into the flat:

'I was rude to Dr Forte, but only because the fact was I was very worried and I wasn't getting satisfaction from him, until in the end I lost my temper. I thought, "this is useless", which I shouldn't have done, but I couldn't help it. And I felt awful because, I thought, "he hasn't got where he is today through nothing". But he wasn't doing me any good. Can you understand what I'm trying to say? To me, he was useless. All he kept telling me was that Eddie's trouble was nerves, and I knew it weren't nerves. I mean, no-one don't go paralysed through nerves. And I think this is what – and after a couple of days of him coming home and then on the Friday, when it happened again, this is when it got to the stage of me thinking, "If he comes in my door I shall tell him to get out".'

It is not possible adequately to portray the variety of experience of doctors and of people's reactions to their experience in this small section of a chapter; to do so would require presenting the material from the interviews at much too great a length. The distinctive characteristics of the private accounts are that they are highly idiosyncratic and personal. In contrast with the uniformity of the generally respectful attitudes and the hierarchical ordering of the different parts of the health service according to the scientific status of the problems they deal with, the private accounts are highly fragmented and are no respecters of hierarchies.

Conclusion

This conclusion takes the discussion full circle, back to the initial observations concerning the difference between Stimson's and Webb's findings (1975) and the findings in the present study. It was said earlier that the explanation for the much more assertive and critical stance which Stimson and Webb report people adopting might have been a function of the group dynamic in the discussion organized by the researchers, which legitimated people's private accounts. If this is true, then we might conclude that were the people involved in the present study to be brought together in a group, they, too, might make public their private stories of doctors and health services. The fragmentation and lack of coherence in the private accounts in the interviews seems to indicate that the dominance of medical ideology over common-sense attitudes is such that it is not possible for individuals to make sense of their personal experience of health services on their own. When they discuss their relationship with doctors and health services, the significance of their personal experience becomes lost and is often (if not always) made redundant. However, in the context where individuals discuss their experiences of doctors and health services together in a group, it is possible for them to endorse and thus legitimate each other's experiences and these will then be incorporated into their public accounts.

One further point remains, and that is a reiteration of the observation from previous chapters that 'experts" own definitions make a significant contribution to the commonsense attitudes and values of public accounts. In this case, the observation is especially important because it demonstrates the significance of the medical contribution to commonsense. An important, but unintended, consequence of that contribution is that, in absorbing the ideas and values of the dominant sections of the medical profession, lay people have learned to under-value preventive and community services which are exactly the parts of the health services that official health policy is now attempting to promote.

8 Conclusion

This study set out to investigate the meaning of the terms 'health' and 'illness' to a particular group of individuals. The choice of research methods was made on the basis of a number of assumptions about the way in which 'ordinary' people (i.e., people without medical qualifications) think about their health. The first and most important assumption was that the relationship people have to health and illness is governed by commonsense ideas and values which are grounded in their way of life. To the extent that this is true, those commonsense ideas and values ought not to be taken out of context and studied apart from the rest of people's lives. It was assumed that each person's own experience of illness and medical care as well as their knowledge of the experience of their direct and close acquaintances would be part of the fabric of commonsense and ought therefore to be included in the investigation. Finally, the authority of medical science and the medical profession over matters of health and illness is such that it was considered naive not to assume that they affect commonsense ideas about health and illness. However, rather than make an *a priori* judgment about the extent to which medical ideas have been incorporated into the fabric of commonsense, this was left as a matter for empirical verification.

The ethnographic approach the study adopted was chosen because it seemed the most appropriate way to investigate people's lives as a whole, whilst at the same time paying particular attention to their relationship to health and illness. The research methods are outlined in the introductory chapter where their advantages and disadvantages are also considered. Without wanting to re-tread ground which has already been covered, it is worthwhile indicating the positive results achieved using these methods.

In general, the ethnographic approach is one that encourages attention to the detail of people's lives and thus to the differences between individuals. This makes it more rather than less likely that interpretations of ethnographic material will bear witness to the part each person plays in shaping the course of his or her own life without losing sight of the fact that they do so in conditions that are not of their own choosing. This is of special significance in the present context in view of the criticism (in Chapter 1) of approaches in medical sociology to lay people as patients, and particularly of the characterization of ordinary people in the 'medicalization of life' thesis as passive and dependent.

In this study, many of the people who were interviewed shared experiences in common, either because they belonged to the same families and households or simply by virtue of having been brought up in the same small area of London. This made it possible to record different individuals' points of view concerning the same range of subjects. At the same time, the concentration on a relatively small number of people meant that most people could be interviewed more than once, so that it was also possible to discuss the same subject with the same person but at different times. It was through these methods that the variations in the content of the interviews which were eventually identified in terms of the distinction between public as opposed to private accounts, were made apparent.

The discovery of the difference between public and private accounts is of course one of the major analytic themes of the study; the other concerns the process of medicalization as defined in Chapter 5. This conclusion considers the practical implications of both these themes for research into lay health beliefs, for work in the field of health education/promotion and prevention, and for the medical profession.

The argument with respect to the difference between the two types of account can be summarized as follows. Public accounts in general draw attention to aspects of people's experience and to ideas and values that they believe are likely to win 'public' approval (i.e., the approval of the person to whom they are talking). In the words of Douglas (1971) they appeal to the 'lowest common denominator' in public morality. Public accounts of health, illness, and health services do the same thing but have an added dimension which is that they draw attention to aspects of experience, ideas, and values that people believe are acceptable to doctors and compatible with a medical point of view. This is because health and illness are subject to modern, scientific, and medical legitimations – i.e., to medical ideological domination.

Public accounts are selective and partial. In general, they exclude those parts of people's experience and opinions that might be considered unacceptable and not respectable. In matters of health they exclude experiences and opinions that might be considered unacceptable to members of the medical profession, except and unless they are dealing with one of those particular areas that is subject to commonsense rather than medical legitimation (see Chapter 7). The place where medically unacceptable and incompatible opinions and values are stated is in private accounts. Private accounts are thus no less selective and partial than public accounts in the range of experiences or opinions they express. It is no more accurate to evaluate the relationship people in the study have with doctors, for example, purely on the basis of their private accounts of their contact with doctors, than it is to rely exclusively on public accounts.

The implication of the distinction between the two types of account for empirical research, and particularly for studies of lay health beliefs, is that it is important to know what kind of account the subjects of such studies are giving. The way the researcher can establish this is to experiment with different research methods and techniques of interviewing, or failing that, to be explicit about the possible effect of the method on the study findings and about the way he or she was perceived by people taking part in the research. The key issue in this respect is to what extent the researcher is likely to be seen as some kind of 'expert'?

The discussion in Chapter 5 and 6 shows that in both public and private accounts the commonsense ideas and theories which govern the relationship people in the study have with health, illness, and health services are grounded in their way of life. Chapter 5 established a powerful similarity between the moral significances of work and health which carried over into the analysis of aetiological theories in Chapter 6. For example, the two main public theories of the causes of illness (e.g., the 'external/unavoidable/no blame' and 'internal/unavoidable/no blame' combinations of categories) replicated exactly the theory of natural inequality as the basis of social hierarchies (outlined in Chapter 3). There were also powerful similarities in the attitude of mind that people were expected to have in relation to both work and health. The private accounts of episodes of illness and the private aetiological theories showed that for people in the study there is no clear separation between illness and what is happening in the rest of their lives. The way in which they respond to feeling unwell is determined as much by their position in the sexual division of labour and at work as anything else, and they see illness as the product of the particular set of circumstances in which the person finds him or herself.

This analysis has some practical implications for health education/promotion and preventive health work. It suggests two things. First, that changes in commonsense ideas and theories about health and illness (and thus in health-related behaviour) are not likely to occur in the absence of changes in other areas of people's lives. It may therefore be more important to change people's position in relation to employment, for example, or to change the sexual division of labour, than constantly to direct attention to health attitudes and beliefs. Second, public health/health education campaigns might be more effective if they were addressed to specific groups of people or to people in specific sets of social circumstances rather than the public as a whole.

Finally, the analysis of the process of medicalization in previous chapters suggests that the medical profession makes an important contribution to commonsense ideas about health and illness, although not always in ways that are intended. Notably, it has been suggested that people learn the values they attach to the different parts of the health service (e.g., hospitals as opposed to primary care or the community and preventive health services) from the medical profession. The symbolic ordering of the different parts of the service in matters of prestige and the quality of buildings and equipment is not lost on patients, and no-one wants to feel that the service they are getting is second-class or second-rate. It follows from this that a re-ordering of the medical profession's own priorities so that the community and preventive services are made more prestigious might make an important – although not necessarily an immediate – impact on public consciousness.

References

Armstrong, D. (1979) The emancipation of biographical medicine. *Social Science and Medicine* **13A**: 1–8.

Bailey, F. G. (ed.) (1971) *Gifts and Poison: the Politics of Reputation*. Oxford: Basil Blackwell.

Balint, M. (1957) *The Doctor, his Patient and the Illness*. Tonbridge Wells: Pitman Medical Co.

Barnes, J. A. (1969a) Graph theory and social networks: a technical comment on connectedness and connectivity. *Sociology* **3**: 215–32.

_____ (1969b) Networks and political process. In Mitchell, J. Clyde (ed.), *Social Networks in Urban Situations: analyses of personal relationships in central African towns*. Manchester: Manchester University Press.

Barrett, M. and Roberts, H. (1978) Doctors and their patients. The social control of women in general practice. In Smart, C. and Smart, B. (eds.), *Women, Sexuality and Social Control*. London: Routledge & Kegan Paul.

Bell, C. and Newby, H. (1972) *Community Studies. An Introduction to the Sociology of the Local Community*. London: Allen & Unwin.

Blaxter, M. and Paterson, E. with assistance of Sheila Murray (1982) *Mothers and Daughters: a three generational study of health attitudes and behaviour*. London: Heinemann Educational Books.

_____ (1983) The goodness is out of it: the meaning of food to two generations. In Murcott, A. (ed.), *The Sociology of Food and Eating*. Aldershot: Gower.

Bott, E. (1957) *Family and Social Network. Roles, norms and external relationships in ordinary urban families*. London: Tavistock. (Revised edition, 1971).

British Medical Association (1970) *Primary Medical Care*. Planning Unit Report No.4. London: B.M.A.

Busfield, J. (1974) Ideologies and Reproduction. In Richards, M. P. M. (ed.), *The Integration of a Child into the Social World*. London: Cambridge University Press.

Calder, A. L. R. (1969) *The People's War 1939-45*. London: Cape.

Cartwright, A. (1967) *Patients and their Doctors. A study of general practice*. London: Routledge & Kegan Paul.

Castells, M. (1976) Is there an urban sociology? and Theory and ideology in urban sociology. In Pickvance, C. G. (ed.), *Urban Sociology: critical essays*. London: Tavistock Publications.

City and East London Area Health Authority (T) (1975) *Primary Health Care*.

_____ (1976a) *Documents commenting on 'Priorities for Health and Social Services' and 'Resource Allocation Working Party Report'*.

_____ (1976b) *Accident and Emergency Services*.

Cockburn, C. (1977) *The Local State. Management of Cities and People*. London: Pluto Press.

Cowie, B. (1976) The cardiac patient's perception of his heart attack. *Social Science and Medicine* **10**: 87-96.

Crawford, R. (1977) You are dangerous to your health: the ideology and politics of victim blaming. *International Journal of Health Services* **7** (4): 663-680.

Davis, A. and Horobin, G. (eds.) (1977) *Medical Encounters: the experience of illness and treatment*. London: Croom Helm.

Davis, F. (1960) Uncertainty in medical prognosis, clinical and functional. *American Journal of Sociology* **66**: 41-47.

_____ (1963) *Passage through Crisis: Polio victims and their families*. Indianapolis: Bobbs-Merrill.

Deakin, M. and Ungerson, C. (1977) Leaving London: *Planned Mobility and the Inner City*. London: Heinemann, for the Centre for Environmental Studies.

Dennis, N., Henriques, F., Slaughter, C. (1969) *Coal is our Life. An analysis of a Yorkshire mining community*. London: Tavistock Publications.

Dennis, R. (1978) Decline of manufacturing employment in Greater London: 1966-74. *Urban Studies* **15**: 63-73.

Department of Health and Social Security (1976a) *Sharing Resources for Health in England*. Report of the Resource Allocation Working Party. London: HMSO.

_____ (1976b) *Priorities for Health and Personal Social Services in England: a consultative document*. London: HMSO.

_____ (1976c) *Prevention and Health: Everybody's Business: a reassessment of public and personal health.* London: HMSO.

_____ (1979) *Patients First: A consultative paper on the structure and management of the National Health Service in England and Wales.* London: HMSO.

Dingwall, R. (1976) *Aspects of Illness.* London: Martin Robertson.

Donnison, D. V., Chapman, V., Meacher, M., Sears, A., and Urwin K. (1965) *Social Policy and Administration. Studies in the development of social services at the local level.* London: Allen & Unwin.

Douglas, J. D. (1971) *American Social Order: Social rules in a pluralistic society.* New York: Free Press.

Ehrenreich, B. and Ehrenreich, J. (1978) Medicine and social control. In Ehrenreich, J. (ed.), *The Cultural Crisis of Modern Medicine.* New York: Monthly Review Press.

Ehrenreich, B. and English, D. (1973) *Witches, Midwives and Nurses.* Glass Mountain Pamphlets. New York: The Feminist Press.

Eisenberg, L. (1977) Disease and Illness: distinctions between professional and popular ideas of sickness. *Culture, Medicine and Psychiatry* **1**: 9–23.

Figlio, K. (1978) Chlorosis and chronic disease in nineteenth century Britain: the social construction of somatic illness in a capitalist society. *Social History* **3**: No 2.

Finlayson, A. and McEwen, J. (1977) *Coronary Heart Disease and Patterns of Living.* London: Croom Helm.

Frankenberg, R. (1976) In the production of their lives, men(?) . . . Sex and gender in British community studies. In Barker, D. L. and Allen, S. (eds.), *Sexual Divisions and Society: process and change.* London: Tavistock Publications.

Freidson, E. (1961) *Patients' Views of Medical Practice: A study of subscribers to a prepaid medical plan in the Bronx.* New York: Russell Sage Foundation.

_____ (1970) *Profession of Medicine: A study of the sociology of applied knowledge.* New York: Dodd, Mead & Co

_____ (1972) Disability as social deviance. In Freidson, E. and Lorber, J. (eds.), *Medical Men and their Work.* Chicago: Aldine Atherton.

Friend, A. and Metcalfe, A. (1981) *Slump City: the politics of mass unemployment.* London: Pluto Press.

Galtung, J. (1969) *Theory and Methods of Social Research* London: Allen & Unwin.

Gardner, J. (1976) Political economy of domestic labour in capitalist society. In Barker, D. L. and Allen, S. (eds.), *Dependence and Exploitation in Work and Marriage*. Harlow: Longman.

Giddens, A. (1976) *New Rules of Sociological Method: A positive critique of interpretative sociologies*. London: Hutchinson.

Gittins, D. (1982) *Fair Sex: Family Size and Structure 1900-39*. London: Hutchinson University Library.

Glaser, B. and Strauss, A. (1965) *Awareness of Dying*. Chicago: Aldine.

Glass, R. and Frenkel, M. (1946) *A Profile of Bethnal Green*. Association for Planning and Regional Reconstruction, 24 Gordon Square, London.

Goffman, E. (1959) *The Presentation of Self in Everyday Life*. Garden City, New York: Doubleday & Co.

Goldthorpe, J. H., Lockwood, D., Bechhoffer, F., and Platt, J. (1968) *The Affluent Worker: industrial attitudes and behaviour*. London: Cambridge University Press.

Graham, H. (1979) Prevention and health: every mother's business. A comment on child health policies in the 1970s. In Harris, C. (ed.), *The Sociology of the Family: New directions for Britain*. Sociological Review Monograph 28: Keele.

Habermas, J. (1971) *Toward a Rational Society. Student protest, science and politics*. London: Heinemann.

Hall, P. (ed.) (1981) *The Inner City in Context*. London: Heinemann.

Harris, C. C. (1969) *The Family. An Introduction*. London: Allen & Unwin.

Harrison, T. (1976) *Living through the Blitz*. London: Collins.

Helman, C. (1978) Feed a Cold, Starve a Fever: Folk models of infection in an English suburban community, and their relation to medical treatment. *Culture, Medicine and Psychiatry* **2**: 107-137.

Herzlich, C. (1973) *Health and Illness: a social psychological analysis*. London: Academic Press.

Honigsbaum, F. (1979) *The Division in British Medicine: A history of the separation of general practice from hospital care 1911-1968*. London: Kogan Page Ltd.

Horwitz, A. (1977) Social networks and pathways to psychiatric treatment. *Social Forces* **56**: 86-105.

Howick, C. and Key, T. (1978) *The Local Economy of Tower Hamlets: An Inner City profile*. Centre for Environmental

Studies Research Series, 26.

Hunt, J. and Hunt, A. (1974) Marxism and the family. *Marxism Today* February: 59–64.

Illich, I. (1976) *Limits to Medicine*. London: Calders & Boyars Ltd.

Kadushin, C. (1966) The friends and supporters of psychotherapy: on social circles in urban life. *American Sociological Review* **31**: 786–802.

Knox, P. L. (1979) Medical deprivation, area deprivation and public policy. *Social Science and Medicine* **13D**: 111–21.

Laslett, B. and Rapoport, R. (1975) Collaborative interviewing and interactive research. *Journal of Marriage and the Family* **37**: 968–77.

Littlejohn, J. (1963) *Westrigg: The Sociology of a Cheviot Parish*. London: Routledge & Kegan Paul.

London Borough of Tower Hamlets (1978) *Planning in West Bethnal Green*. Planning Department.

McKee, L. (1982) Fathers' participation in infant care: a critique. In McKee, L. and O'Brien, M. (eds.), *The Father Figure*. London: Tavistock Publications.

McKee, L. and O'Brien, M. (1982) *The Father Figure*. London: Tavistock Publications.

McKinlay, J. B. (1970) A brief description of a study on the utilization of maternity and child welfare facilities by a lower working-class subculture. *Social Science and Medicine* **4**: 551–56.

—— (1973) Social networks, lay consultation and help-seeking behaviour. *Social Forces* **51**: 275–92.

Marris, P. (1974) *Loss and Change*. London: Routledge & Kegan Paul.

Mitchell, J. Clyde (1969) The concept and use of social networks. In Mitchell, J. Clyde (ed.), *Social Networks in Urban Situations: analyses of personal relationships in central African towns*. Manchester: Manchester University Press.

—— (1983) Case and situation analysis. *The Sociological Review* **31** (2): 187–211.

Morgan, D. H. J. (1975) *Social Theory and the Family*. London: Routledge & Kegan Paul.

Morpeth, R. and Langton, P. (1974) Contemporary matriarchies: women alone – independent or incomplete? *Cambridge Anthropology* **1**: No 3.

Myers, M. (1975) Urban deprivation and the G.L.C. *Greater*

London Intelligence Quarterly No 31: 21–31.

Navarro, V. (1977) *Medicine Under Capitalism*. London: Croom Helm.

Oakley, A. (1974) *The Sociology of Housework*. London: Martin Robertson.

_____ (1980) *Women Confined: towards a sociology of child-birth*. Oxford: Martin Robertson.

_____ (1981) Interviewing women: a contradiction in terms. In Roberts, H. (ed.) *Doing Feminist Research*. London: Routledge & Kegan Paul.

Parsons, T. (1951) *The Social System*. New York: Free Press.

Parsons, T. and Fox, R. (1968) Illness, therapy and the modern urban Amercian family. In Bell, N. W. and Vogel, E. F. (eds.), *A Modern Introduction to the Family*. New York: Free Press.

Pilisuk, M. and Froland, C. (1978) Kinship, social networks, social support and health. *Social Science and Medicine* **12B**: 273–80.

Pill, R. and Stott, N. C. H. (1982) Concepts of illness causation and responsibility: some preliminary data from a sample of working class mothers. *Social Science and Medicine* **16**: 43–52.

Price, F. V. (1981) Only connect? Issues in charting social networks. *The Sociological Review* **29** (2): 283–312.

Richardson, S. A., Dohrenwend, B. S., and Klein, D. (1965) *Interviewing - Its Forms and Functions*. New York: Basic Books.

Roberts, R. (1971) *The Classic Slum. Salford life in the first quarter of the century*. Manchester: Manchester University Press.

Robinson, D. (1971) *The Process of Becoming Ill*. London: Routledge & Kegan Paul.

Royal College of General Practitioners (1977) *Trends in General Practice*. Fry, J. (ed.). London: British Medical Journal.

Salzberger, R. C. (1976) Cancer: assumptions and reality concerning delay, ignorance and fear. In Loudon, J. B. (ed.), *Social Anthropology and Medicine*, ASA Monograph 13. London: Academic Press.

Selltiz, C., Jahoda, M., Deutsch, M., and Cook, S. (1965) *Research Methods in Social Relations*. Rinehard & Winston: New York.

Sennett, R. (1980) *Authority*. London: Martin Secker & Warburg Ltd.

Shankland, G., Willmott, P. and Jordan, D. (1977) *Inner London: policies for dispersal and balance*. HMSO: London.

Sjoberg, G. and Nett, R. (1968) *A Methodology for Social Research*. New York: Harper & Row.

Skrimshire, A. (1978) *Area Disadvantage, Social Class and the Health Service*. Social Evaluation Unit, Oxford, in association with Canning Town Community Development Project.

Stacey, M. (1960) *Tradition and Change: A study of Banbury*. London: Oxford University Press.

Stedman Jones, G. (1971) *Outcast London: A study in the relationship between classes in Victorian society*. Oxford: Clarendon Press.

Stevens, R. (1966) *Medical Practice in Modern England. The impact of specialization and State medicine*. New York and London: Yale University Press.

Stimson, G. and Webb, B. (1975) *Going to See the Doctor: the consultation process in general practice*. London: Routledge & Kegan Paul.

Strong, P. M. (1979a) Sociological imperialism and the profession of medicine: a critical examination of the thesis of medical imperialism. *Social Science and Medicine* **13A**: 199–215.

―――― (1979b) *The Ceremonial Order of the Clinic: parents, doctors and medical bureaucracies*. London: Routledge & Kegan Paul.

Sudnow, D. (1967) *Passing On: the social organization of dying*. Englewood Cliffs: Prentice Hall Inc.

Syson, L. and Young, M. (1974) Poverty in Bethnal Green. In Young, M. (ed.), *Poverty Report 1974*. London: Maurice Temple Smith Ltd.

Townsend, P. (1957) *The Family Life of Old People. An inquiry in East London*. London: Routledge & Kegan Paul.

―――― (1974) Inequality and the Health Service. *Lancet* **1**: 1179–189.

Townsend, P. and Davidson, N. (1982) *Inequalities in Health. The Black Report*. Harmondsworth: Penguin Books.

Tudor Hart, J. (1971) Inverse care law. *Lancet* **(i)**: 405–412.

Voysey, M. (1975) *A Constant Burden: the reconstitution of family life*. London: Routledge & Kegan Paul.

Waitzkin, H. (1979) Medicine, superstructure and micropolitics. *Social Science and Medicine* **13A**: 601–609.

Williams, Raymond (1973) *The Country and the City*. London: Chatto & Windus.

Williams, Rory (1983) Concepts of health: an analysis of lay logic.

Sociology **17** (2): 185–205.

Willmott, Peter and Young, M. (1971) *Family and Class in a London Suburb*. London: New English Library.

Willmott, Phyllis (1979) *Growing up in a London Village: Family life between the wars*. London: Peter Owen Ltd.

Young, M. (1955) A Study of the Extended Family in East London. Ph.d. thesis submitted at London University.

Young, M. and Willmott, P. (1957) *Family and Kinship in East London*. London: Routledge & Kegan Paul.

Yudkin, J. (1978) Changing patterns of resource allocation in a London Teaching district. *British Medical Journal* **2**: 1212–1215.

Zola, I. K. (1978) Medicine as an institution of social control. In Ehrenreich, J. (ed.) *The Cultural Crisis of Modern Medicine*. New York: Monthly Review Press.

Name Index

The names of the people who took part in the study are to be found in the subject index.

Subject Index